PCOS DIET COOKBOOK FOR WEIGHT LOSS

DELICOUS RECIPES FOR MANAGING POLYCYSTIC OVARIAN SYNDROME, BALANCING HORMONES AND BOOSTING FERTILITY.

MARIA G. KYLE
DOROTHY MATA

Copyright (c) 2024 MARIA G. KYLE

AND DORATHY MATA

All rights reserved. No part of this publication may be reproduced, distributed, or transmitted in any form or by any means, including photocopying, recording, or other electronic or mechanical methods, without the prior written permission of the publisher, except in the case of brief quotations embodied in critical reviews and certain other noncommercial uses permitted by copyright law.

Table of Contents

- INTRODUCTION 5
  - Understanding PCOS 5
  - The Role of Diet in Managing PCOS 7
- CHAPTER TWO 12
  - PRINCIPLES OF THE PCOS DIET 12
    - Key Nutritional Guidelines For Managing PCOS ... 12
    - Foods to Include and Avoid 16
    - Importance of Fiber, Protein and Healthy Fats 18
- CHAPTER THREE 20
  - BREAKFAST RECIPES 20
    - Healthy Quinoa Breakfast Bowl 20
    - Greek Yogurt Parfait with Berries 22
    - Spinach and Feta Egg Muffins 24
    - Chia Seed Pudding With Almond Milk 26
    - Smoothie Recipes For Hormone Balance 28
- CHAPTER FOUR 39
  - LUNCH AND DINNER RECIPES 39
    - Grilled Salmon with quinoa and asparagus 39
    - Turkey and Vegetable Stir Fry 42
    - Lentil and Sweet Potato Curry 44
    - Zucchini Noodles with pesto and Cherry Tomatoes 47
- CHAPTER FIVE 51

SNACKS AND SMALL BITES 51
    Hummus and Veggies Platter 53
    Almond Butter Energy Balls 55
    Greek Yogurt Deep With Fresh Veggies 57
    Roasted Chickpeas With Spices 59
    Greek Yogurt with Berries 61
    Apple Slices with Almond Butter 63
    Mixed Nuts Snack 65
    Hard-Boiled Eggs 67
    Chia Seed Pudding 69
    Caprese Skewers 71
    Cottage Cheese with Pineapple 73
    Smoked Salmon Cucumber Bites 75
    Quinoa Salad Cups 77
    Trail Mix 80
    Edamame 82
    Stuffed Bell Peppers 83

CHAPTER SIX 88
  DESSERTS AND SWEET TREAT 88
    Berry and Coconut Milk Smoothie Bowl 88
    Dark Chocolate Avocado Mousse 90
    Baked Apples with Cinnamon and Walnuts 92
    Greek Yogurt with Honey and Berries 94

- Chia Seed Pudding with Mango 95
- Banana Oatmeal Cookies 97
- Lemon Blueberry Yogurt Parfait 99
- Coconut Macaroons 101
- Peanut Butter Banana Smoothie 103
- Mango Coconut Rice Pudding 104

CHAPTER SEVEN 106
MEAL PLANNING TIPS AND SAMPLE MENUS . 106
- How To Plan Meals for PCOS 106
- Sample Weekly Meal Plans 109
- Tips for Grocery Shopping and Batch Cooking 117

CHAPTER EIGHT 122
LIFESTYLE TIPS FOR MANAGING PCOS 122
- Importance of Exercise 122
- Stress Management Techniques 127
- Sleep and PCOS 131

CHAPTER NINE 135
RESOURCES AND FURTHER READING 135
- Recommended Books and Websites 135
- Support Groups and Online Communities 139

CONCLUSION 143

INTRODUCTION

Understanding PCOS

Polycystic Ovary Syndrome (PCOS) is a multifaceted health condition that presents a spectrum of symptoms and challenges for women of reproductive age. It is estimated that PCOS affects between 8–13% of women in this age group, making it one of the most common hormonal disorders worldwide. Despite its prevalence, a significant number of cases remain undiagnosed, which can lead to a delay in treatment and management of the syndrome.

PCOS is characterized by a combination of symptoms that can include irregular menstrual cycles, infertility, hirsutism (excessive hair growth), acne, and obesity. These symptoms are a result of hormonal imbalances in the body, particularly an excess of androgens, which are typically considered male hormones. Women with PCOS may also experience insulin resistance, which can increase the risk of developing type 2 diabetes, hypertension, and cardiovascular diseases.

The diagnosis of PCOS is based on the Rotterdam criteria, which require two out of three key features: hyperandrogenism, ovulatory dysfunction, and polycystic ovaries visible on ultrasound. However, the presentation of PCOS can vary significantly from one individual to another, making it a complex condition to diagnose and treat.

The management of PCOS is equally diverse and includes lifestyle modifications such as diet and exercise to improve insulin sensitivity and achieve weight loss if necessary. Medical treatments may involve hormonal contraceptives to regulate menstrual cycles, anti-androgens to reduce hair growth and acne, and fertility medications for those seeking to become pregnant.

Understanding PCOS is not only crucial for those directly affected by the condition but also for healthcare providers, as it requires a multidisciplinary approach to care. This includes support from gynecologists, endocrinologists, dermatologists, dietitians, and mental health professionals. Education and awareness about PCOS can empower women to seek the help they need and can lead to better health outcomes.

The Role of Diet in Managing PCOS

Diet plays a crucial role in managing Polycystic Ovary Syndrome (PCOS), a hormonal disorder that affects many women of reproductive age. The condition is often accompanied by insulin resistance, which can exacerbate symptoms such as weight gain, irregular menstrual cycles, and infertility. By adopting a mindful and balanced diet, women with PCOS can improve their hormonal balance, increase insulin sensitivity, and alleviate some of the condition's most challenging symptoms.

A well-structured PCOS diet focuses on several key principles:

Low Glycemic Index (GI) Foods: Consuming foods with a low GI can help maintain stable blood sugar levels, which is essential for managing insulin resistance—a common issue in PCOS.

Balanced Macronutrients: A diet with an appropriate balance of carbohydrates, proteins, and fats can support overall health and hormone regulation.

Fiber-Rich Foods: High-fiber foods can aid digestion, reduce insulin spikes, and promote a feeling of fullness, helping to manage weight.

Anti-Inflammatory Foods: Chronic inflammation is linked to PCOS, so incorporating anti-inflammatory foods like leafy greens, nuts, and fatty fish can be beneficial.

Antioxidants: Foods rich in antioxidants can help combat oxidative stress, which is also associated with PCOS.

Nutrient-Dense Foods and Hormone Balance

Choosing nutrient-dense foods is essential for women with PCOS to support hormone balance and overall health. Adequate intake of vitamins and minerals, such as vitamin D, magnesium, and zinc, is crucial as deficiencies in these nutrients have been linked to worsened PCOS symptoms. Vitamin D, for example, plays a role in insulin sensitivity and may help regulate menstrual cycles. Magnesium is involved in hundreds of biochemical reactions in the body, including those related to insulin and glucose metabolism. Zinc is important for ovarian function and hormone regulation. Incorporating a variety of colorful fruits and vegetables provides a wide range of antioxidants, phytochemicals, and fiber that can help reduce inflammation, support immune function, and promote gut health—all of which are beneficial for managing PCOS symptoms.

It's important to note that while dietary changes can have a positive impact, they should be part of a comprehensive management plan that includes regular physical activity, stress reduction, and medical treatment when necessary.

Remember, managing PCOS is a personal journey, and what works for one person may not work for another. It's about finding the right balance that suits your body and lifestyle while addressing the specific challenges of PCOS.

How This Cookbook Can Help

Embarking on the journey of managing PCOS can be overwhelming, but this cookbook is designed to be a beacon of guidance and support. It provides a curated collection of recipes that are not only delicious but also specifically tailored to address the unique dietary needs of those with PCOS. The cookbook aims to simplify the process of making healthier food choices that can have a positive impact on managing the condition.

The recipes in this cookbook are carefully crafted to:

Regulate Insulin Levels: With a focus on low-glycemic index foods, the recipes help in stabilizing blood sugar levels, which is crucial for reducing insulin resistance—a common challenge in PCOS.

Reduce Inflammation: Chronic inflammation is linked to many of the symptoms of PCOS. The anti-inflammatory recipes aim to soothe and reduce inflammation, promoting a healthier body environment.

Balance Hormones: Hormonal imbalance is at the core of PCOS. The meals are designed to provide the right nutrients that support hormonal health and balance.

Improve Fertility: For those looking to boost fertility, the cookbook includes recipes that focus on nutrients known to support reproductive health.

Support Weight Management: Many individuals with PCOS struggle with weight issues. The recipes are mindful of calorie content and nutritional balance, aiding in weight management efforts.

Enhance Overall Well-being: Beyond addressing PCOS symptoms, the cookbook promotes an overall healthier lifestyle, which can improve energy levels, mood, and general well-being.

This cookbook serves as a practical tool, offering easy-to-follow recipes that bring clarity and enjoyment to the process of meal preparation. It's a companion for those who seek to regain control over their PCOS symptoms through the power of nourishing, wholesome food.

For anyone navigating the complexities of PCOS, this cookbook is more than just a collection of recipes—it's a roadmap to a healthier, more balanced life. It's about transforming the kitchen into a place of healing and hope, where every meal is a step towards better health.

CHAPTER TWO

PRINCIPLES OF THE PCOS DIET

Key Nutritional Guidelines For Managing PCOS

Effective management of PCOS through diet involves focusing on nutrient-dense foods that support hormone balance, regulate insulin levels, and promote overall well-being. Start by prioritizing complex carbohydrates such as whole grains (oats, quinoa, whole wheat), which are rich in fiber and help stabilize blood sugar levels. Incorporate lean protein sources like chicken, turkey, fish, tofu, and legumes to support muscle maintenance and hormone synthesis. Healthy fats from sources such as avocados, nuts (like almonds, walnuts), seeds (flaxseeds, chia seeds), and olive oil are essential for hormone production and reducing inflammation. Aim for a balanced intake of these macronutrients throughout the day to maintain steady energy levels and prevent cravings. Additionally, include plenty of fiber-rich foods like fruits, vegetables, legumes, and whole grains to support digestive health and promote satiety. Limit refined carbohydrates and sugars found in processed foods, sweets, and sugary beverages, as these can contribute to insulin resistance and weight gain. Choose omega-3 fatty acids from fatty fish (salmon, trout), flaxseeds, and walnuts to reduce inflammation and improve insulin sensitivity. Hydration is also crucial—drink plenty of water throughout the day to support digestion and detoxification processes. Practice portion control and balanced meals, spacing regular meals evenly throughout the day and incorporating healthy snacks as needed to maintain stable blood sugar levels. By following these nutritional guidelines, women with PCOS can effectively manage symptoms, support fertility, and reduce long-term health risks associated with the condition.

These guidelines are crafted to empower individuals with PCOS to make informed dietary choices that positively impact their health and well-being, providing a foundation for managing the complex interplay of hormonal and metabolic factors characteristic of PCOS. These guidelines includes:

1. **Balanced Macronutrients:** Aim for a balanced intake of macronutrients—carbohydrates, proteins, and fats. Choose complex carbohydrates such as whole grains (oats, quinoa, whole wheat), which are high in fiber and help stabilize blood sugar levels. Include lean proteins like chicken, turkey, fish, tofu, and legumes, which support muscle maintenance and hormone synthesis. Incorporate healthy fats from sources like avocados, nuts, seeds, and olive oil, which aid in hormone production and reduce inflammation.

2. **Fiber-Rich Foods:** Include plenty of fiber in your diet from fruits, vegetables, legumes, and whole grains. Fiber helps

regulate blood sugar levels, promotes satiety, and supports digestive health. Aim for at least 25 grams of fiber per day, focusing on a variety of sources to maximize nutrient intake and benefit gut health.

3. **Moderate and Balanced Carbohydrate Intake:** Manage carbohydrate intake by choosing complex carbohydrates over simple sugars. Limit refined carbohydrates and sugars found in processed foods, sweets, sugary beverages, and white bread. Instead, opt for whole grains, vegetables, and fruits, which provide sustained energy and minimize blood sugar spikes.

4. **Healthy Protein Choices:** Opt for lean protein sources such as poultry, fish, tofu, tempeh, and legumes. Protein is essential for muscle maintenance, hormone synthesis, and promoting satiety. Spread protein intake evenly throughout the day to support stable energy levels and prevent cravings.

5. **Healthy Fats:** Incorporate sources of healthy fats, including avocados, nuts (such as almonds, walnuts), seeds (flaxseeds, chia seeds), and olive oil. These fats support hormone production, reduce inflammation, and aid in nutrient absorption. Limit saturated fats and trans fats found in fried foods, processed snacks, and fatty cuts of meat.

6. **Omega-3 Fatty Acids:** Include omega-3 fatty acids, found in fatty fish (salmon, trout, sardines), flaxseeds, chia seeds, and walnuts. Omega-3s help reduce inflammation, improve insulin sensitivity, and support cardiovascular health. Aim to consume fatty fish at least twice a week or consider a high-quality omega-3 supplement.

7. **Limited Added Sugars and Processed Foods:** Minimize intake of added sugars, sugary snacks, and processed foods, as these can contribute to insulin resistance, weight gain, and inflammation. Read food labels carefully and choose natural sweeteners like honey or maple syrup in moderation, if needed.

8. **Hydration:** Stay well-hydrated by drinking plenty of water throughout the day. Water supports digestion, helps maintain energy levels, and aids in detoxification processes. Limit intake of sugary beverages and caffeinated drinks, which can disrupt blood sugar levels and hydration balance.

9. **Portion Control and Balanced Meals:** Practice portion control and aim for balanced meals that include a combination of carbohydrates, proteins, and fats. Eating balanced meals helps regulate blood sugar levels, prevents energy dips, and supports overall metabolic health.

10. **Regular Meals and Snacks:** Establish regular eating patterns with meals spaced evenly throughout the day. Include healthy snacks between meals to maintain stable blood sugar levels and prevent overeating. Opt for nutrient-dense snacks such as yogurt with berries, whole grain crackers with hummus, or a handful of nuts and seeds.

Foods to Include and Avoid

To effectively manage PCOS, it's essential to focus on a balanced diet that supports hormone regulation, improves insulin sensitivity, and promotes overall health. Include nutrient-dense foods that are rich in vitamins, minerals, fiber, and healthy fats. Opt for complex carbohydrates such as whole grains (like oats, quinoa, brown rice) which provide sustained energy and help stabilize blood sugar levels. Lean proteins from sources like poultry, fish, tofu, and legumes are important for muscle maintenance and hormone synthesis. Healthy fats found in avocados, nuts (such as almonds, walnuts), seeds (like flaxseeds, chia seeds), and olive oil contribute to hormone balance and reduce inflammation. Include plenty of fiber-rich foods such as fruits, vegetables, and legumes to support digestive health and promote satiety.

It's also crucial to incorporate foods rich in omega-3 fatty acids, such as fatty fish (salmon, mackerel, sardines), flaxseeds, and walnuts, as these fats have been shown to reduce inflammation and improve insulin sensitivity. Hydration is key—drink plenty of water throughout the day to support metabolic processes and overall well-being.

On the other hand, it's important to limit or avoid certain foods that can exacerbate symptoms of PCOS. Minimize intake of refined carbohydrates, sugary snacks, and beverages with added sugars, as these can lead to rapid spikes in blood sugar levels and worsen insulin resistance. Processed foods high in trans fats and saturated fats, like fried foods, baked goods, and fatty meats, should also be reduced, as they contribute to inflammation and metabolic dysfunction. Dairy and meat products that are high in hormones or antibiotics should be consumed in moderation or sourced from organic, hormone-free options when possible.

By adopting a diet focused on whole, nutrient-dense foods while limiting processed and inflammatory foods, individuals with PCOS can effectively manage symptoms, support hormone balance, and reduce the risk of long-term health complications associated with the condition. These dietary principles provide a foundation for improving overall health outcomes and enhancing quality of life for women living with PCOS.

Importance of Fiber, Protein and Healthy Fats

Fiber plays a critical role in managing PCOS by stabilizing blood sugar levels, promoting satiety, and supporting digestive health. Incorporating adequate fiber from sources such as whole grains (like oats, quinoa, and whole wheat), fruits, vegetables, and legumes helps prevent rapid spikes and crashes in blood glucose, which is particularly beneficial for individuals with insulin resistance commonly associated with PCOS. Additionally, fiber supports gut health by promoting regular bowel movements and reducing the risk of constipation, which can alleviate discomfort and support overall well-being.

Protein is essential for women with PCOS to support muscle maintenance, hormone synthesis, and satiety. Lean protein sources such as poultry, fish, tofu, and legumes provide amino acids necessary for tissue repair and hormone production. Including protein in each meal and snack helps regulate appetite, stabilize blood sugar levels, and prevent cravings for unhealthy foods, thus supporting weight management—a key concern for many women with PCOS.

Healthy fats are another crucial component of a PCOS-friendly diet as they support hormone balance, reduce inflammation, and aid in the absorption of fat-soluble vitamins. Sources of healthy fats include avocados, nuts (such as almonds, walnuts), seeds (like flaxseeds, chia seeds), and olive oil. Omega-3 fatty acids, found in fatty fish (salmon, mackerel, sardines), flaxseeds, and walnuts, have been shown to specifically benefit women with PCOS by improving insulin sensitivity, reducing androgen levels, and supporting cardiovascular health. Incorporating a variety of healthy fats in moderation helps maintain cell structure, regulate hormone production, and reduce inflammation—a cornerstone of managing the hormonal imbalances associated with PCOS.

By prioritizing fiber-rich foods, lean proteins, and healthy fats, women with PCOS can effectively support hormone balance, manage insulin resistance, and promote overall health and well-being. These dietary components not only provide essential nutrients but also contribute to sustainable weight management and improved metabolic outcomes, offering a holistic approach to managing the multifaceted challenges of PCOS.

CHAPTER THREE

BREAKFAST RECIPES

Healthy Quinoa Breakfast Bowl

Ingredients:
- 1/2 cup quinoa, rinsed
- 1 cup water or almond milk (unsweetened)
- 1/2 teaspoon ground cinnamon
- 1 tablespoon honey or maple syrup (optional, for sweetness)
- 1/2 cup mixed berries (such as strawberries, blueberries, raspberries)
- 1 small banana, sliced
- 2 tablespoons chopped nuts (such as almonds, walnuts, or pecans)
- 1 tablespoon chia seeds
- 1/4 cup Greek yogurt or coconut yogurt (unsweetened)
- Fresh mint leaves, for garnish (optional)

Instructions:

1. Cook the Quinoa:
   - In a small saucepan, combine the quinoa and water or almond milk. Bring to a boil over medium-high heat.
   - Reduce the heat to low, cover, and simmer for about 15 minutes, or until the quinoa is cooked and the liquid is absorbed.

- Remove from heat and let it sit covered for 5 minutes. Fluff the quinoa with a fork and stir in ground cinnamon and honey or maple syrup, if using.

2. Assemble the Breakfast Bowl:
    - Divide the cooked quinoa into serving bowls.
    - Top each bowl with mixed berries, sliced banana, chopped nuts, and chia seeds.

3. Add Yogurt and Garnish:
    - Spoon Greek yogurt or coconut yogurt over each bowl.
    - Garnish with fresh mint leaves, if desired.

4. Serve and Enjoy!
    - Mix everything together gently just before eating to combine the flavors and textures.

Greek Yogurt Parfait with Berries

Ingredients:
- 1 cup Greek yogurt (plain, unsweetened)
- 1 cup mixed berries (such as strawberries, blueberries, raspberries)
- 1/4 cup granola (choose a variety with low added sugars)
- 1 tablespoon honey or maple syrup (optional, for sweetness)
- Fresh mint leaves, for garnish (optional)

Instructions:

1. Prepare the Berries:
   - Wash and dry the mixed berries. If using strawberries, hull and slice them into bite-sized pieces.

2. Assemble the Parfait:
   - In a glass or bowl, start with a layer of Greek yogurt at the bottom.
   - Add a layer of mixed berries on top of the yogurt.
   - Sprinkle a layer of granola over the berries.

3. Repeat Layers:
   - Repeat the layers until you reach the top of the glass or bowl, ending with a layer of berries and granola.

4. Drizzle with Sweetener (Optional):
   - If desired, drizzle honey or maple syrup over the top layer for added sweetness.

5. Garnish and Serve:
   - Garnish with fresh mint leaves for a refreshing touch.

6. Enjoy Your Greek Yogurt Parfait
   - Serve immediately and enjoy this nutritious and delicious parfait as a satisfying breakfast or snack.

Spinach and Feta Egg Muffins

Ingredients:
- 6 large eggs
- 1 cup fresh spinach, chopped
- 1/2 cup crumbled feta cheese
- 1/4 cup milk (regular or almond milk)
- 1/4 teaspoon garlic powder
- Salt and pepper, to taste
- Cooking spray or olive oil, for greasing muffin tin

Instructions:

1. Preheat Oven and Prepare Muffin Tin:
   - Preheat your oven to 350°F (175°C). Grease a 12-cup muffin tin with cooking spray or olive oil to prevent sticking.

2. Prepare Egg Mixture:
   - In a large mixing bowl, crack the eggs and whisk them together with milk until well combined.
   - Stir in chopped spinach, crumbled feta cheese, garlic powder, salt, and pepper. Mix until all ingredients are evenly distributed.

3. Fill Muffin Cups:
   - Pour the egg mixture evenly into the prepared muffin tin, filling each cup about 3/4 full.

4. Bake:

- Place the muffin tin in the preheated oven and bake for 20-25 minutes, or until the egg muffins are set and lightly golden on top. They should puff up and a toothpick inserted into the center should come out clean.

5. Cool and Serve:
   - Remove the egg muffins from the oven and let them cool in the muffin tin for a few minutes.
   - Carefully remove the egg muffins from the tin and transfer them to a wire rack to cool completely.

6. Enjoy Your Spinach and Feta Egg Muffins!
   - Serve the egg muffins warm or at room temperature. They can be stored in an airtight container in the refrigerator for up to 3 days. They are perfect for a quick and nutritious breakfast or snack on the go!

Chia Seed Pudding With Almond Milk

Ingredients:
- 1/4 cup chia seeds
- 1 cup almond milk (unsweetened)
- 1 tablespoon maple syrup or honey (optional, for sweetness)
- 1/2 teaspoon vanilla extract
- Fresh berries or fruit, for topping (optional)
- Nuts or seeds, for topping (optional)

Instructions:

1. Mix Ingredients:
   - In a mixing bowl or glass jar, combine the chia seeds, almond milk, maple syrup or honey (if using), and vanilla extract. Stir well to combine all ingredients thoroughly.

2. Let It Sit:
   - Cover the bowl or jar and refrigerate for at least 2 hours, or preferably overnight. This allows the chia seeds to absorb the liquid and form a pudding-like consistency.

3. Stir Occasionally:
   - After the first 30 minutes, stir the mixture again to prevent clumping and ensure even distribution of chia seeds.

4. Serve:
   - Once the chia seeds have absorbed the liquid and the mixture has thickened to a pudding consistency, remove from the refrigerator.

- Stir the pudding to break up any clumps that may have formed.

5. Add Toppings (Optional):
   - Serve the chia seed pudding in individual bowls or jars.
   - Top with fresh berries or fruit, nuts, or seeds for added texture and flavor.

6. Enjoy Your Chia Seed Pudding with Almond Milk!
   - Serve chilled and enjoy this nutritious and satisfying pudding as a breakfast, snack, or dessert option.

Smoothie Recipes For Hormone Balance

Smoothies can be an excellent addition to your diet for supporting hormone balance, offering a convenient way to pack in essential nutrients. For a hormone-balancing smoothie, try blending together a mix of antioxidant-rich berries like strawberries and blueberries, which help combat inflammation and oxidative stress that can disrupt hormone production. Add a tablespoon of ground flaxseeds or chia seeds to provide omega-3 fatty acids and fiber, crucial for hormone synthesis and digestive health. Including a source of healthy fats such as almond butter or avocado helps stabilize blood sugar levels and supports hormone production. For a creamy texture and added protein, consider adding unsweetened almond milk or coconut milk along with a scoop of protein powder, either plant-based or collagen.

Here is a list of five basic smoothies for hormone balancing and their recipes:
Certainly! Here's a recipe for a Berry Bliss Hormone-Balancing Smoothie:

Berry Bliss Hormone-Balancing Smoothie

Ingredients:
- 1 cup mixed berries (such as strawberries, blueberries, raspberries)
- 1 cup spinach
- 1/2 avocado
- 1 tablespoon almond butter

- 1 tablespoon chia seeds
- 1 cup unsweetened almond milk or coconut water
- Optional: 1 tablespoon honey or maple syrup (for added sweetness)

Instructions:

1. Prepare Ingredients:
   - Wash the berries and spinach thoroughly. If using strawberries, remove the hulls.
   - Pit and scoop out the flesh of the avocado.

2. Blend Ingredients:
   - In a blender, combine the mixed berries, spinach, avocado, almond butter, chia seeds, and almond milk (or coconut water).
   - Optional: Add honey or maple syrup for sweetness, if desired.

3. Blend Until Smooth:
   - Blend on high speed until the mixture is smooth and creamy. Add more almond milk or coconut water if needed to reach your desired consistency.

4. Serve:
   - Pour the smoothie into a glass.
   - Optionally, garnish with a few extra berries or a sprinkle of chia seeds on top.

5. Enjoy Your Berry Bliss Hormone-Balancing Smoothie!

- Serve immediately and enjoy this nutritious and delicious smoothie that supports hormone balance and overall well-being.

Benefits: This smoothie is rich in antioxidants from the mixed berries, which help combat inflammation and oxidative stress that can disrupt hormone balance.

Green Goddess Hormone-Balancing Smoothie

Ingredients:
- 1 cup spinach
- 1 cup kale, chopped
- 1/2 cucumber, peeled and chopped
- 1/2 cup pineapple chunks (fresh or frozen)
- Juice of 1/2 lemon
- 1 tablespoon fresh ginger, grated
- 1 cup coconut water or water
- Optional: 1 tablespoon hemp seeds or flaxseeds

Instructions:

1. Prepare Ingredients:
   - Wash the spinach and kale thoroughly. Chop the kale into smaller pieces.
   - Peel and chop the cucumber.
   - Juice half a lemon and grate the fresh ginger.

2. Blend Ingredients:
   - In a blender, combine the spinach, kale, cucumber, pineapple chunks, lemon juice, grated ginger, and coconut water (or water).
   - Optional: Add hemp seeds or flaxseeds for added fiber and omega-3 fatty acids.

3. Blend Until Smooth:

- Blend on high speed until the mixture is smooth and creamy. Add more water or coconut water if needed to reach your desired consistency.

4. Serve:
   - Pour the smoothie into glasses.
   - Optionally, garnish with a slice of cucumber or a sprinkle of hemp seeds on top.

5. Enjoy Your Green Goddess Hormone-Balancing Smoothie!
   - Serve immediately and enjoy this refreshing and nutritious smoothie that supports hormone balance and overall well-being.

Benefits: This smoothie is packed with nutrient-dense ingredients. Spinach and kale provide essential vitamins and minerals that support hormone production and overall health.

Chocolate Almond Butter Hormone-Balancing Smoothie

Ingredients:
- 1 cup almond milk (unsweetened)
- 1 tablespoon almond butter
- 1 tablespoon cacao powder (unsweetened)
- 1/2 banana
- 1 cup spinach
- 1 tablespoon chia seeds
- Optional: 1 scoop protein powder (plant-based or collagen)
- Optional: 1 tablespoon honey or maple syrup (for added sweetness)

Instructions:

1. Prepare Ingredients:
   - Peel and slice the banana.
   - Wash the spinach thoroughly.

2. Blend Ingredients:
   - In a blender, combine almond milk, almond butter, cacao powder, banana, spinach, chia seeds, and protein powder (if using).
   - Optional: Add honey or maple syrup for added sweetness, if desired.

3. Blend Until Smooth:
   - Blend on high speed until the mixture is smooth and creamy. Adjust the consistency by adding more almond milk if needed.

4. Serve:
   - Pour the smoothie into glasses.
   - Optionally, garnish with a sprinkle of cacao nibs or a drizzle of almond butter on top.

5. Enjoy Your Chocolate Almond Butter Hormone-Balancing Smoothie!
   - Serve immediately and enjoy this indulgent yet nutritious smoothie that supports hormone balance and overall well-being.

Benefits: This smoothie combines the richness of almond butter and cacao powder, providing healthy fats, antioxidants, and minerals like magnesium and zinc that support hormone production and mood regulation.

Turmeric Mango Hormone-Balancing Smoothie

Ingredients:
- 1 cup mango chunks (fresh or frozen)
- 1/2 banana
- 1/2 teaspoon turmeric powder (or 1 teaspoon grated fresh turmeric)
- 1/2 teaspoon grated ginger
- 1 cup coconut milk (unsweetened)
- 1 tablespoon hemp seeds or flaxseeds
- Optional: 1 tablespoon honey or maple syrup (for added sweetness)

Instructions:

1. Prepare Ingredients:
   - Peel and chop the mango and banana.
   - Grate the fresh turmeric and ginger.

2. Blend Ingredients:
   - In a blender, combine mango chunks, banana, turmeric powder (or grated turmeric), grated ginger, coconut milk, and hemp seeds or flaxseeds.
   - Optional: Add honey or maple syrup for added sweetness, if desired.

3. Blend Until Smooth:
   - Blend on high speed until the mixture is smooth and creamy. Adjust the consistency by adding more coconut milk if needed.

4. Serve:

   - Pour the smoothie into glasses.

   - Optionally, garnish with a slice of mango or a sprinkle of turmeric powder on top.

5. Enjoy Your Turmeric Mango Hormone-Balancing Smoothie!

   - Serve immediately and enjoy this vibrant and nutrient-packed smoothie that supports hormone balance and overall well-being.

Benefits: This smoothie combines the tropical sweetness of mango with the anti-inflammatory properties of turmeric and ginger, which can help reduce inflammation and support hormone balance.

Berry Avocado Chia Hormone-Balancing Smoothie

Ingredients:
- 1 cup mixed berries (such as strawberries, blueberries, raspberries)
- 1/2 avocado
- 1 tablespoon chia seeds
- 1/2 cup Greek yogurt (plain, unsweetened)
- 1 cup unsweetened almond milk or coconut water
- Optional: 1 tablespoon honey or maple syrup (for added sweetness)

Instructions:

1. Prepare Ingredients:
   - Wash the mixed berries thoroughly. If using strawberries, remove the hulls.
   - Pit and scoop out the flesh of the avocado.

2. Blend Ingredients:
   - In a blender, combine mixed berries, avocado, chia seeds, Greek yogurt, and almond milk (or coconut water).
   - Optional: Add honey or maple syrup for added sweetness, if desired.

3. Blend Until Smooth:
   - Blend on high speed until the mixture is smooth and creamy. Adjust the consistency by adding more almond milk or coconut water if needed.

4. Serve:
   - Pour the smoothie into glasses.
   - Optionally, garnish with a few extra berries or a sprinkle of chia seeds on top.

5. Enjoy Your Berry Avocado Chia Hormone-Balancing Smoothie!
   - Serve immediately and enjoy this creamy and nutrient-rich smoothie that supports hormone balance and overall well-being.

Benefits: Greek yogurt provides probiotics that support gut health, which is crucial for hormone balance. Optional honey or maple syrup adds sweetness without compromising the health benefits.

CHAPTER FOUR

LUNCH AND DINNER RECIPES

Grilled Salmon with quinoa and asparagus

Ingredients:
- 2 salmon filets (about 6 ounces each), skin-on
- 1 cup quinoa, rinsed
- 1 bunch asparagus, tough ends trimmed
- 2 tablespoons olive oil
- 2 cloves garlic, minced
- 1 lemon, divided
- Salt and pepper, to taste
- Fresh herbs (such as parsley or dill), chopped, for garnish

Instructions:

1. Prepare Quinoa:
   - In a medium saucepan, bring 2 cups of water to a boil. Add the rinsed quinoa and a pinch of salt. Reduce heat to low, cover, and simmer for about 15 minutes, or until quinoa is cooked and water is absorbed. Fluff with a fork and set aside.

2. Preheat Grill:
   - Preheat your grill to medium-high heat.

3. Prepare Asparagus:
   - Place the trimmed asparagus spears on a baking sheet. Drizzle with 1 tablespoon of olive oil, minced garlic, juice of half a lemon, salt, and pepper. Toss to coat evenly.

4. Grill Asparagus:
   - Grill the asparagus over medium-high heat for about 5-7 minutes, turning occasionally, until tender and lightly charred. Remove from the grill and set aside.

5. Grill Salmon:
   - Rub the salmon filets with the remaining tablespoon of olive oil. Season generously with salt and pepper.
   - Place the salmon filets on the grill, skin-side down. Grill for about 4-5 minutes per side, depending on thickness, until the salmon is cooked through and easily flakes with a fork.

6. Serve:
   - Divide the cooked quinoa among serving plates. Top with grilled salmon filets and grilled asparagus.
   - Drizzle with the juice of the remaining half lemon.
   - Garnish with chopped fresh herbs, such as parsley or dill.

7. Enjoy Your Grilled Salmon with Quinoa and Asparagus!
   - Serve immediately and enjoy this nutritious and flavorful dish.

Tips:
- You can marinate the salmon filets in a mixture of olive oil, lemon juice, garlic, and herbs for 30 minutes before grilling for added flavor.

- Feel free to customize by adding additional vegetables or herbs to the quinoa or asparagus.

Turkey and Vegetable Stir Fry

Ingredients:

- 1 lb turkey breast or turkey tenderloin, thinly sliced
- 2 cups mixed vegetables (such as bell peppers, broccoli, snap peas, carrots)
- 2 tablespoons soy sauce (or tamari for gluten-free option)
- 1 tablespoon oyster sauce (optional)
- 1 tablespoon sesame oil
- 2 cloves garlic, minced
- 1-inch piece of ginger, grated
- 2 green onions, chopped
- 1 tablespoon cornstarch mixed with 2 tablespoons water (optional, for thickening sauce)
- Cooked rice or quinoa, for serving
- Sesame seeds, for garnish (optional)

Instructions:

1. Prepare the Turkey:
   - Heat 1 tablespoon of sesame oil in a large skillet or wok over medium-high heat.
   - Add the thinly sliced turkey and stir-fry until cooked through and lightly browned. Remove from the skillet and set aside.

2. Stir-Fry Vegetables:
   - In the same skillet or wok, add a little more sesame oil if needed.

- Add minced garlic and grated ginger. Stir-fry for about 30 seconds until fragrant.

3. Add Mixed Vegetables:
 - Add the mixed vegetables to the skillet. Stir-fry for 3-5 minutes, or until vegetables are crisp-tender.

4. Combine Turkey and Sauce:
 - Return the cooked turkey to the skillet with the vegetables.
 - Add soy sauce (or tamari), oyster sauce (if using), and chopped green onions. Stir to combine well.

5. Thicken Sauce (Optional):
 - If desired, stir in the cornstarch mixture to thicken the sauce. Cook for another minute until the sauce has thickened and coats the turkey and vegetables.

6. Serve:
 - Serve the turkey and vegetable stir-fry hot over cooked rice or quinoa.
 - Garnish with sesame seeds and additional chopped green onions, if desired.

7. Enjoy Your Turkey and Vegetable Stir-Fry!
 - Serve immediately and enjoy this flavorful and nutritious dish.

Tips:
- You can customize the vegetables based on what you have on hand or your preferences.
- Feel free to add additional spices or chili flakes for extra heat.

Lentil and Sweet Potato Curry

Ingredients:

- 1 cup dried lentils (green or brown), rinsed
- 2 medium sweet potatoes, peeled and diced
- 1 onion, chopped
- 3 cloves garlic, minced
- 1 tablespoon fresh ginger, grated
- 1 can (14 oz) diced tomatoes
- 1 can (14 oz) coconut milk
- 2 tablespoons curry powder
- 1 teaspoon ground turmeric
- 1 teaspoon ground cumin
- 1/2 teaspoon cayenne pepper (adjust to taste, optional)
- Salt and pepper, to taste
- 2 tablespoons coconut oil or vegetable oil
- Fresh cilantro, chopped, for garnish
- Cooked rice or naan bread, for serving

Instructions:

1. Prepare Lentils:
   - In a large pot, bring 3 cups of water to a boil. Add the rinsed lentils and reduce heat to low. Simmer for about 20-25 minutes, or until lentils are tender. Drain any excess water and set aside.

2. Cook Sweet Potatoes:
   - While the lentils are cooking, heat coconut oil or vegetable oil in a large skillet or pot over medium heat.

- Add chopped onion and sauté for 3-4 minutes, until softened.

- Stir in minced garlic and grated ginger. Sauté for another minute until fragrant.

- Add diced sweet potatoes to the skillet. Cook for 5-7 minutes, stirring occasionally, until sweet potatoes begin to soften.

3. Add Spices and Tomatoes:

- Sprinkle curry powder, ground turmeric, ground cumin, and cayenne pepper (if using) over the sweet potatoes and onions. Stir to coat the vegetables with the spices.

- Add diced tomatoes (with their juices) to the skillet. Stir well to combine.

4. Simmer Curry:

- Pour in the coconut milk and cooked lentils. Stir to combine all ingredients.

- Season with salt and pepper to taste.

- Bring the mixture to a simmer, then reduce heat to low. Cover and simmer for 15-20 minutes, or until sweet potatoes are tender and flavors have melded together.

5. Serve:

- Serve the lentil and sweet potato curry hot over cooked rice or with naan bread.

- Garnish with fresh chopped cilantro.

6. Enjoy Your Lentil and Sweet Potato Curry!

- Serve immediately and enjoy this hearty and flavorful curry dish.

Tips:

- Adjust the spice level by adding more or less cayenne pepper, depending on your preference.
- You can substitute canned lentils for dried lentils to save time, adjusting cooking times accordingly.
- This curry can be stored in the refrigerator for up to 3 days, making it a great option for meal prep.

Zucchini Noodles with pesto and Cherry Tomatoes

Ingredients:

- 4 medium zucchinis
- 1 cup cherry tomatoes, halved
- 1/2 cup basil pesto (store-bought or homemade)
- 2 tablespoons olive oil
- 2 cloves garlic, minced
- Salt and pepper, to taste
- Grated Parmesan cheese, for serving (optional)
- Fresh basil leaves, chopped, for garnish

Instructions:

1. Prepare Zucchini Noodles:
   - Using a spiralizer, spiralize the zucchini into noodles. Alternatively, you can use a vegetable peeler to create long, thin strips resembling noodles.

2. Cook Cherry Tomatoes:
   - Heat olive oil in a large skillet over medium heat.
   - Add minced garlic and cook for 1 minute until fragrant.
   - Add halved cherry tomatoes to the skillet. Cook for 2-3 minutes, stirring occasionally, until tomatoes start to soften and release their juices.

3. Add Zucchini Noodles:
   - Add the zucchini noodles to the skillet with the cherry tomatoes and garlic.

- Toss gently using tongs or a spatula to combine. Cook for 2-3 minutes, stirring occasionally, until zucchini noodles are just tender but still crisp.

4. Combine with Pesto:
   - Add basil pesto to the skillet with the zucchini noodles and cherry tomatoes.
   - Toss everything together until the zucchini noodles are evenly coated with the pesto sauce. Remove from heat.

5. Serve:
   - Divide the zucchini noodles with pesto and cherry tomatoes among serving plates.
   - Optionally, garnish with grated Parmesan cheese and chopped fresh basil leaves.

6. Enjoy Your Zucchini Noodles with Pesto and Cherry Tomatoes!
   - Serve immediately and enjoy this light and flavorful dish.

Tips:
- If you prefer softer zucchini noodles, cook them for an additional 1-2 minutes in the skillet.
- Feel free to add grilled chicken, shrimp, or tofu for added protein.

- Chicken and Vegetable Soup

Ingredients:
- 1 lb boneless, skinless chicken breasts or thighs, diced
- 1 onion, chopped
- 2 carrots, peeled and sliced

- 2 celery stalks, sliced
- 2 garlic cloves, minced
- 1 teaspoon dried thyme
- 1 teaspoon dried oregano
- 6 cups chicken broth (low sodium)
- 1 can (14 oz) diced tomatoes, drained
- 1 cup green beans, trimmed and cut into 1-inch pieces
- 1 cup corn kernels (fresh, frozen, or canned)
- Salt and pepper, to taste
- Fresh parsley, chopped, for garnish

Instructions:

1. Cook Chicken:
   - In a large pot or Dutch oven, heat olive oil over medium-high heat.
   - Add diced chicken pieces and cook until browned on all sides, about 5-7 minutes. Remove chicken from the pot and set aside.

2. Sauté Vegetables:
   - In the same pot, add chopped onion, sliced carrots, and sliced celery. Cook for 5 minutes, stirring occasionally, until vegetables begin to soften.
   - Add minced garlic, dried thyme, and dried oregano. Cook for 1 minute until fragrant.

3. Simmer Soup:
   - Return the cooked chicken to the pot.
   - Pour in chicken broth and diced tomatoes (drained). Stir to combine.

- Bring the soup to a boil, then reduce heat to low. Cover and simmer for 20-25 minutes, or until vegetables are tender and chicken is cooked through.

4. Add Green Beans and Corn:
   - Stir in green beans and corn kernels.
   - Cook for an additional 5-7 minutes, until the green beans are tender.

5. Season and Serve:
   - Season the soup with salt and pepper, to taste.
   - Serve hot, garnished with chopped fresh parsley.

6. Enjoy Your Chicken and Vegetable Soup!
   - Serve immediately and enjoy this hearty and comforting soup.

Tips:
- Feel free to add other vegetables such as peas, bell peppers, or spinach according to your preference.
- For a thicker soup, you can stir in a slurry of cornstarch and water during the last few minutes of cooking.
- Store leftovers in an airtight container in the refrigerator for up to 3 days, or freeze for longer storage.

CHAPTER FIVE

SNACKS AND SMALL BITES

Avocado Toast With Whole Grain Bread

Ingredients:
- 2 slices of whole grain bread
- 1 ripe avocado
- 1 tablespoon lemon juice
- Salt and pepper, to taste
- Optional toppings: sliced cherry tomatoes, red pepper flakes, microgreens, or a drizzle of balsamic glaze

Instructions:
1. Toast the whole grain bread slices until golden and crispy.

2. While the bread is toasting, cut the avocado in half and remove the pit. Scoop out the flesh into a bowl.

3. Mash the avocado with a fork until smooth or leave it slightly chunky, according to your preference.

4. Stir in lemon juice, salt, and pepper to taste.

5. Spread the mashed avocado evenly onto the toasted whole grain bread slices.

6. Optional: Top with sliced cherry tomatoes, a sprinkle of red pepper flakes, microgreens, or a drizzle of balsamic glaze for added flavor and texture.

7. Serve immediately and enjoy your classic avocado toast!

Hummus and Veggies Platter

Ingredients:
- 1 cup hummus (store-bought or homemade)
- Assorted fresh vegetables, such as:
  - Carrot sticks
  - Cucumber slices
  - Bell pepper strips (red, yellow, or green)
  - Cherry tomatoes
  - Celery sticks
  - Radishes, thinly sliced
- Optional additions: olives, pickles, pita bread or whole grain crackers

Instructions:

1. Prepare the Hummus:
   - If making homemade hummus, prepare it according to your favorite recipe or use store-bought hummus.

2. Prepare the Vegetables:
   - Wash and prepare the vegetables by cutting them into sticks, slices, or bite-sized pieces.

3. Assemble the Platter:
   - Arrange the hummus in the center of a large serving platter or a shallow bowl.

4. Surround with Vegetables:

- Arrange the assorted fresh vegetables around the hummus, creating an attractive display.

5. Add Optional Additions:
  - Optional: Garnish the platter with olives, pickles, and serve with pita bread or whole grain crackers on the side.

6. Serve:
  - Serve the hummus and veggie platter immediately, and enjoy dipping the vegetables into the creamy hummus.

Tips:
- Customize the platter with your favorite vegetables or add additional dips like tzatziki or guacamole.
- This platter is perfect for gatherings, parties, or as a healthy snack option.

Almond Butter Energy Balls

Ingredients:

- 1 cup rolled oats
- 1/2 cup almond butter (or any nut butter of your choice)
- 1/4 cup honey or maple syrup
- 1/4 cup ground flaxseed
- 1/4 cup mini chocolate chips (optional)
- 1 teaspoon vanilla extract
- Pinch of salt (optional)
- Additional coatings: shredded coconut, cocoa powder, chopped nuts (optional)

Instructions:

1. Combine Ingredients:
   - In a large mixing bowl, combine rolled oats, almond butter, honey or maple syrup, ground flaxseed, mini chocolate chips (if using), vanilla extract, and a pinch of salt (if desired).

2. Mix Thoroughly:
   - Stir the ingredients together until well combined. The mixture should be sticky enough to hold together when rolled into balls.

3. Form Energy Balls:
   - Using a tablespoon or small cookie scoop, scoop out portions of the mixture and roll between your palms to form smooth balls.

4. Optional Coatings:
 - Roll the energy balls in shredded coconut, cocoa powder, or chopped nuts for additional flavor and texture.

5. Chill:
 - Place the energy balls on a baking sheet lined with parchment paper. Chill in the refrigerator for at least 30 minutes to firm up.

6. Store and Enjoy:
 - Once chilled, transfer the almond butter energy balls to an airtight container.
 - Store in the refrigerator for up to 2 weeks, or freeze for longer storage.

7. Serve:
 - Serve the almond butter energy balls chilled as a quick and nutritious snack or energy boost throughout the day.

Tips:
- Customize the energy balls by adding dried fruit like cranberries or raisins, or seeds like chia or hemp seeds.
- Adjust the sweetness by varying the amount of honey or maple syrup according to your preference.
- These energy balls are perfect for on-the-go snacking, pre-workout fuel, or as a healthy treat after meals.

Greek Yogurt Deep With Fresh Veggies

Ingredients:

- 1 cup Greek yogurt (plain, unsweetened)
- 1/2 cucumber, peeled, seeded, and finely diced
- 1/2 red bell pepper, finely diced
- 1/4 cup finely chopped fresh herbs (such as dill, parsley, or chives)
- 1 tablespoon lemon juice
- 1 clove garlic, minced
- Salt and pepper, to taste
- Assorted fresh vegetables for serving (carrot sticks, cucumber slices, bell pepper strips, cherry tomatoes, celery sticks, etc.)

Instructions:

1. Prepare the Greek Yogurt Dip:
   - In a medium mixing bowl, combine Greek yogurt, diced cucumber, diced red bell pepper, finely chopped fresh herbs, lemon juice, minced garlic, salt, and pepper.

2. Mix Thoroughly:
   - Stir all the ingredients together until well combined. Adjust seasoning with salt and pepper to taste.

3. Chill:
   - Cover the bowl and refrigerate the Greek yogurt dip for at least 30 minutes to allow the flavors to meld together.

4. Prepare Fresh Vegetables:

- While the dip is chilling, prepare the assorted fresh vegetables for serving by washing and cutting them into sticks, slices, or bite-sized pieces.

5. Serve:
   - Transfer the chilled Greek yogurt dip to a serving bowl or platter.
   - Arrange the assorted fresh vegetables around the dip for dipping.

6. Enjoy Your Greek Yogurt Dip with Fresh Veggies!
   - Serve immediately as a healthy and refreshing appetizer, snack, or party dip.

Tips:
- Customize the dip by adding other finely chopped vegetables such as cherry tomatoes, green onions, or shredded carrots.
- This dip can be made ahead of time and stored in the refrigerator for up to 3 days.

Roasted Chickpeas With Spices

Ingredients:
- 1 can (15 oz) chickpeas (garbanzo beans), drained, rinsed, and patted dry
- 1 tablespoon olive oil
- 1 teaspoon ground cumin
- 1 teaspoon smoked paprika
- 1/2 teaspoon ground coriander
- 1/2 teaspoon garlic powder
- 1/4 teaspoon cayenne pepper (adjust to taste for spiciness)
- Salt, to taste

Instructions:

1. Preheat Oven:
   - Preheat your oven to 400°F (200°C).

2. Prepare Chickpeas:
   - Drain and rinse the chickpeas thoroughly. Pat them dry using a clean kitchen towel or paper towels to remove excess moisture.

3. Season Chickpeas:
   - In a mixing bowl, toss the chickpeas with olive oil, ground cumin, smoked paprika, ground coriander, garlic powder, cayenne pepper, and salt. Ensure the chickpeas are evenly coated with the spices.

4. Roast Chickpeas:

- Spread the seasoned chickpeas in a single layer on a baking sheet lined with parchment paper or a silicone baking mat.

5. Bake:
   - Bake in the preheated oven for 25-30 minutes, shaking the pan halfway through baking, until the chickpeas are crispy and golden brown.

6. Cool and Serve:
   - Remove from the oven and let the roasted chickpeas cool on the baking sheet for a few minutes before serving.

7. Enjoy Your Roasted Chickpeas with Spices!
   - Serve the roasted chickpeas as a crunchy and flavorful snack or appetizer.

Tips:
- Customize the spices according to your taste preferences. You can add more or less cayenne pepper for spiciness, or try different spice blends like curry powder or chili powder.
- Store any leftovers in an airtight container at room temperature for up to 3 days. Re-crisp them in the oven for a few minutes before serving if needed.

Greek Yogurt with Berries

Ingredients:
- 1 cup Greek yogurt (plain, unsweetened)
- 1/2 cup mixed berries (such as strawberries, blueberries, raspberries)
- 1 tablespoon honey or maple syrup (optional, for sweetness)
- Fresh mint leaves, for garnish (optional)

Instructions:

1. Prepare the Berries:
   - Wash and gently pat dry the mixed berries. If using strawberries, hull and slice them into smaller pieces if desired.

2. Sweeten the Yogurt (Optional):
   - In a small bowl, mix Greek yogurt with honey or maple syrup, if using, until well combined. Adjust sweetness according to your preference.

3. Assemble:
   - Spoon the sweetened Greek yogurt into serving bowls or glasses.

4. Top with Berries:
   - Arrange the mixed berries on top of the Greek yogurt.

5. Garnish (Optional):
   - Garnish with fresh mint leaves for a pop of color and added freshness.

6. Serve:

 - Serve immediately and enjoy your Greek yogurt with berries as a nutritious breakfast, snack, or dessert.

Tips:

- You can customize this recipe by using your favorite type of Greek yogurt (regular, low-fat, or non-fat) and adjusting the amount of honey or maple syrup for sweetness.
- Experiment with different types of berries or add other fruits such as sliced bananas or kiwi for variety.
- Greek yogurt provides protein, probiotics, and calcium, while berries offer antioxidants and vitamins, making this a healthy and satisfying treat.

Apple Slices with Almond Butter

Ingredients:

- 1-2 medium-sized apples (such as Gala, Fuji, or Honeycrisp)
- Almond butter (or any nut butter of your choice)
- Optional toppings: honey, cinnamon, chopped nuts, or granola

Instructions:

1. Prepare the Apples:
   - Wash and dry the apples thoroughly. Core the apples and slice them into thin rounds or wedges.

2. Serve with Almond Butter:
   - Spread a generous amount of almond butter onto each apple slice.

3. Optional Toppings:
   - Drizzle with honey, sprinkle with cinnamon, or add chopped nuts or granola on top of the almond butter for added flavor and texture.

4. Enjoy Your Apple Slices with Almond Butter!
   - Serve immediately as a nutritious and satisfying snack.

Tips:
- Choose apples that are crisp and slightly sweet for the best flavor combination with almond butter.

- Adjust the amount of almond butter according to your preference.
- This snack is not only delicious but also provides a good balance of fiber, healthy fats, and natural sweetness from the apples and almond butter.

Mixed Nuts Snack

Ingredients:

- Mixed nuts (such as almonds, walnuts, cashews, pecans, pistachios)
- Optional additions: dried fruits (like cranberries or raisins), dark chocolate chips, or seeds (such as pumpkin seeds)

Instructions

1. Combine Mixed Nuts:
   - In a small bowl or snack container, mix together a variety of nuts according to your preference. You can use equal parts of almonds, walnuts, cashews, pecans, and pistachios, or any combination you like.

2. Optional Additions:
   - Add dried fruits like cranberries or raisins for a touch of sweetness, dark chocolate chips for a bit of indulgence, or seeds such as pumpkin seeds for added crunch and nutrition.

3. Portion Out:
   - Portion out the mixed nuts into small snack-sized containers or bags for convenient grab-and-go portions.

4. Enjoy Your Mixed Nuts Snack!
   - Enjoy the mixed nuts as a quick and nutritious snack between meals, at work, or while on the go.

Tips:

- Customize the mix by adjusting the types and proportions of nuts based on your taste preferences and dietary needs.
- Mixed nuts are rich in healthy fats, protein, and fiber, making them a satisfying and energy-boosting snack option.
- Store any leftover mixed nuts in an airtight container to maintain freshness.

Hard-Boiled Eggs

Ingredients:

- Hard-boiled eggs (as many as desired)

Instructions:

1. Prepare Hard-Boiled Eggs:
   - Place eggs in a single layer in a saucepan and cover with cold water by about 1 inch.
   - Bring water to a boil over medium-high heat.
   - Once boiling, cover the saucepan and remove it from heat.
   - Let the eggs sit in the hot water for about 10-12 minutes for medium-sized eggs (adjust time slightly for smaller or larger eggs).
   - Drain the hot water and transfer the eggs to a bowl of ice water. Let them cool for a few minutes.

2. Peel and Serve:
   - Gently tap the eggs on a hard surface and peel off the shells.
   - Rinse the peeled eggs under cold water to remove any remaining shell pieces.

3. Enjoy Your Hard-Boiled Eggs!
   - Enjoy the hard-boiled eggs plain, or sprinkle with a pinch of salt and pepper if desired.

Tips:

- Hard-boiled eggs are a convenient and nutritious snack option, rich in protein, vitamins, and minerals.
- Store hard-boiled eggs in the refrigerator in their shells for up to one week. Peel them when ready to eat.
- Hard-boiled eggs can be enjoyed on their own, added to salads, or as a protein-packed snack any time of day.

Chia Seed Pudding

Ingredients:

- 1/4 cup chia seeds
- 1 cup almond milk (or any milk of your choice)
- 1 tablespoon honey or maple syrup (optional, for sweetness)
- 1/2 teaspoon vanilla extract
- Fresh berries or sliced fruits, for topping
- Nuts, seeds, or granola, for topping (optional)

Instructions:

1. Mix Chia Seeds and Liquid:
   - In a bowl or jar, combine chia seeds, almond milk (or your preferred milk), honey or maple syrup (if using), and vanilla extract. Stir well to combine.

2. Let it Set:
   - Cover the bowl or jar and refrigerate for at least 2 hours, or preferably overnight. Stir or shake occasionally within the first hour to prevent clumping.

3. Serve:
   - Once the chia seeds have absorbed the liquid and the mixture has thickened to a pudding-like consistency, give it a good stir.

4. Top and Enjoy:
   - Serve the chia seed pudding in bowls or glasses.

- Top with fresh berries or sliced fruits and any additional toppings like nuts, seeds, or granola for added texture and flavor.

5. Enjoy Your Chia Seed Pudding!
   - Enjoy as a healthy and delicious breakfast, snack, or dessert.

Tips:
- Customize your chia seed pudding by adding flavors such as cocoa powder, matcha powder, or cinnamon to the mixture before refrigerating.
- Adjust the sweetness by varying the amount of honey or maple syrup according to your preference.
- Chia seed pudding can be stored in the refrigerator for up to 3-4 days. Stir well before serving if it thickens too much.

Caprese Skewers

Ingredients:

- Cherry or grape tomatoes
- Fresh mozzarella balls (bocconcini)
- Fresh basil leaves
- Balsamic glaze or balsamic reduction, for drizzling (optional)
- Wooden skewers or toothpicks

Instructions:

1. Prepare Ingredients:
   - Rinse the cherry or grape tomatoes and pat them dry.
   - Drain the fresh mozzarella balls (bocconcini) if they are stored in liquid.

2. Assemble Skewers:
   - Thread one cherry tomato, one fresh mozzarella ball (bocconcini), and one fresh basil leaf onto each skewer or toothpick.
   - Repeat until all ingredients are used, adjusting the amount based on the size of your skewers or toothpicks.

3. Drizzle with Balsamic Glaze (Optional):
   - Arrange the Caprese skewers on a serving platter.
   - Optional: Drizzle balsamic glaze or balsamic reduction over the skewers for added flavor. Alternatively, you can serve the balsamic glaze on the side for dipping.

4. Serve:

  - Serve the Caprese skewers immediately as an appetizer or party snack.

Tips:

- Choose ripe cherry or grape tomatoes and fresh mozzarella balls for the best flavor and texture.
- If using wooden skewers, soak them in water for about 15-20 minutes before assembling to prevent them from burning during grilling or broiling.
- Caprese skewers can be prepared ahead of time and stored in the refrigerator until ready to serve. Drizzle with balsamic glaze just before serving for the best presentation.

Cottage Cheese with Pineapple

Ingredients:

- 1 cup cottage cheese (preferably low-fat or full-fat, depending on your preference)
- 1 cup fresh pineapple chunks (or canned pineapple chunks in juice, drained)

Instructions:

1. Prepare Ingredients:
   - If using fresh pineapple, peel and cut it into bite-sized chunks. If using canned pineapple, drain the chunks from the juice.

2. Combine Cottage Cheese and Pineapple:
   - In a serving bowl or plate, spoon the cottage cheese.

3. Add Pineapple:
   - Arrange the pineapple chunks on top of the cottage cheese.

4. Serve:
   - Serve the cottage cheese with pineapple immediately as a nutritious and satisfying snack or light meal.

Tips:
- Customize your cottage cheese with pineapple by adding a sprinkle of cinnamon, a drizzle of honey or maple syrup, or a handful of nuts or seeds for added crunch and flavor.

- Cottage cheese is rich in protein and calcium, while pineapple provides vitamins, minerals, and natural sweetness, making this combination a healthy and balanced snack option.
- Store any leftover cottage cheese with pineapple in an airtight container in the refrigerator for up to 2 days.

Smoked Salmon Cucumber Bites

Ingredients:

- English cucumber, cut into thick rounds
- Smoked salmon slices, cut into smaller pieces
- Cream cheese or Greek yogurt
- Fresh dill, chopped (optional, for garnish)
- Capers (optional, for garnish)

Instructions:

1. Prepare Cucumber Rounds:
   - Wash the English cucumber thoroughly and cut it into thick rounds, about 1/2 inch thick.

2. Assemble Smoked Salmon Bites:
   - Spread a thin layer of cream cheese or Greek yogurt on top of each cucumber round.

3. Add Smoked Salmon:
   - Place a piece of smoked salmon on top of the cream cheese or Greek yogurt.

4. Garnish (Optional):
   - Optional: Sprinkle with chopped fresh dill and add a few capers on top for added flavor and garnish.

5. Serve:
   - Arrange the smoked salmon cucumber bites on a serving platter.

6. Enjoy Your Smoked Salmon Cucumber Bites!
   - Serve immediately as an elegant appetizer or snack.

Tips:
- For a dairy-free option, you can omit the cream cheese or Greek yogurt and simply top the cucumber rounds with smoked salmon.
- Customize the bites by adding a squeeze of lemon juice, a sprinkle of black pepper, or a dash of hot sauce for extra flavor.
- Smoked salmon cucumber bites are not only delicious but also packed with protein and healthy fats, making them a nutritious choice for any occasion.

Quinoa Salad Cups

Ingredients:

- 1 cup quinoa, rinsed
- 2 cups water or vegetable broth
- 1 cucumber, diced
- 1 bell pepper (any color), diced
- 1/2 cup cherry tomatoes, halved
- 1/4 cup red onion, finely chopped
- 1/4 cup fresh parsley or cilantro, chopped
- Juice of 1 lemon
- 3 tablespoons olive oil
- Salt and pepper, to taste
- Optional additions: crumbled feta cheese, avocado slices, roasted chickpeas

Instructions:

1. Cook Quinoa:
   - In a medium saucepan, bring the water or vegetable broth to a boil. Add the rinsed quinoa, reduce heat to low, cover, and simmer for about 15 minutes, or until all liquid is absorbed and quinoa is cooked. Remove from heat and let it cool.

2. Prepare Vegetables:
   - While the quinoa is cooking, prepare the vegetables. Dice the cucumber, bell pepper, cherry tomatoes, and finely chop the red onion and fresh parsley or cilantro.

3. Assemble Salad:

- In a large mixing bowl, combine the cooked and cooled quinoa with the diced cucumber, bell pepper, cherry tomatoes, red onion, and fresh parsley or cilantro.

4. Make Dressing:
- In a small bowl, whisk together the lemon juice, olive oil, salt, and pepper to taste.

5. Combine and Toss:
- Pour the dressing over the quinoa and vegetables. Toss gently until everything is well combined and coated with the dressing.

6. Serve in Cups:
- Spoon the quinoa salad into small cups or bowls for individual servings.

7. Optional Garnishes:
- Optional: Garnish with crumbled feta cheese, avocado slices, or roasted chickpeas for extra flavor and texture.

8. Enjoy Your Quinoa Salad Cups!
- Serve immediately as a delicious and nutritious appetizer or light meal.

Tips:
- Quinoa salad cups can be served immediately or refrigerated for a few hours before serving to allow flavors to meld.
- Customize the salad by adding other vegetables like diced avocado, shredded carrots, or cucumber.

- Quinoa is a complete protein, and this salad is packed with fiber, vitamins, and antioxidants, making it a healthy choice for lunch, dinner, or as a party appetizer.

Trail Mix

Ingredients:

- 1 cup raw almonds
- 1 cup raw cashews
- 1 cup pumpkin seeds (pepitas)
- 1 cup dried cranberries
- 1 cup dark chocolate chips or chunks
- 1 cup unsweetened coconut flakes (optional)
- 1/2 teaspoon sea salt (optional, for a sweet-salty balance)

Instructions:

1. Combine Ingredients:
   - In a large mixing bowl, combine raw almonds, raw cashews, pumpkin seeds (pepitas), dried cranberries, dark chocolate chips or chunks, and unsweetened coconut flakes if using.

2. Mix Well:
   - Stir all the ingredients together until well combined.

3. Optional Seasoning:
   - Optional: Sprinkle sea salt over the mixture for a sweet-salty balance. Adjust to taste.

4. Store:
   - Transfer the trail mix to an airtight container or individual snack bags for portioned servings.

5. Enjoy Your Trail Mix!

- Serve as a convenient and nutritious snack for hiking, travel, or anytime you need an energy boost.

Tips:
- Customize your trail mix by adding other nuts like walnuts or pecans, seeds such as sunflower seeds or chia seeds, or dried fruits like raisins or apricots.
- Keep portions in mind to balance calorie intake, especially if adding chocolate or coconut flakes.
- Trail mix is versatile and can be enjoyed as is or added to yogurt, oatmeal, or salads for extra crunch and flavor.

Edamame

Ingredients:

- 1 cup frozen edamame (in pods)
- Sea salt (optional, for seasoning)

Instructions:

1. Cook Edamame:
   - Bring a pot of water to a boil. Add frozen edamame (still in pods) and cook for about 5 minutes, or until tender.

2. Drain and Season (Optional):
   - Drain the cooked edamame and transfer to a bowl. Sprinkle with sea salt, if desired, and toss to coat evenly.

3. Serve:
   - Serve the edamame immediately as a nutritious and satisfying snack.

Tips:
- Edamame can also be served cold after boiling, making it a refreshing snack option.
- Customize your edamame by adding other seasonings such as garlic powder, sesame seeds, or soy sauce for added flavor.
- Edamame is rich in protein, fiber, and various vitamins and minerals, making it a healthy and filling snack choice.

Stuffed Bell Peppers

Ingredients:
- 4 large bell peppers (any color)
- 1 cup quinoa, cooked
- 1 can (15 oz) black beans, drained and rinsed
- 1 cup corn kernels (fresh or frozen)
- 1 cup diced tomatoes (canned or fresh)
- 1/2 cup shredded cheese (cheddar, mozzarella, or your favorite)
- 1 teaspoon chili powder
- 1/2 teaspoon cumin
- 1/2 teaspoon garlic powder
- Salt and pepper, to taste
- Fresh cilantro or parsley, chopped (for garnish)

Instructions:

1. Prepare Bell Peppers:
   - Preheat your oven to 375°F (190°C). Cut the tops off the bell peppers and remove the seeds and membranes. Rinse them under cold water.

2. Cook Quinoa:
   - In a medium saucepan, cook quinoa according to package instructions. Set aside.

3. Prepare Filling:

- In a large bowl, combine cooked quinoa, black beans, corn kernels, diced tomatoes, shredded cheese, chili powder, cumin, garlic powder, salt, and pepper. Mix well to combine.

4. Stuff Bell Peppers:
   - Stuff each bell pepper with the quinoa mixture, pressing down gently to fill completely.

5. Bake:
   - Place the stuffed bell peppers upright in a baking dish. Cover with foil and bake in the preheated oven for 30-35 minutes, or until the peppers are tender.

6. Optional: Add Cheese (if desired):
   - Remove foil and sprinkle additional cheese on top of each stuffed pepper. Bake uncovered for an additional 5 minutes, or until the cheese is melted and bubbly.

7. Serve:
   - Remove from the oven and let cool slightly. Garnish with chopped cilantro or parsley, if desired.

8. Enjoy Your Stuffed Bell Peppers!
   - Serve hot as a satisfying and nutritious main dish.

Tips:
- You can customize the filling by adding ground turkey, ground beef, or shredded chicken for extra protein.
- Make it vegetarian or vegan by omitting the cheese or using vegan cheese alternatives.

- Stuffed bell peppers can be stored in the refrigerator for up to 3-4 days. Reheat in the microwave or oven before serving.

Rice Cake with Avocado and Tomato

Ingredients:

- Rice cakes (choose your favorite variety)
- 1 ripe avocado
- 1-2 tomatoes, thinly sliced
- Salt and pepper, to taste
- Optional toppings: red pepper flakes, fresh basil leaves, balsamic glaze

Instructions:

1. Prepare Ingredients:
   - Slice the avocado in half, remove the pit, and scoop out the flesh. Mash it lightly with a fork and season with salt and pepper to taste.

2. Assemble Rice Cakes:
   - Spread a generous layer of mashed avocado onto each rice cake.

3. Add Tomato Slices:
   - Arrange thinly sliced tomatoes on top of the mashed avocado layer.

4. Season:
   - Sprinkle with additional salt and pepper if desired. You can also add a pinch of red pepper flakes for a bit of heat.

5. Optional Garnish:

- Garnish with fresh basil leaves or drizzle with balsamic glaze for added flavor and presentation.

6. Serve:
   - Serve the rice cakes with avocado and tomato immediately as a light and nutritious snack or appetizer.

Tips:
- Choose whole grain rice cakes for added fiber and nutrition.
- Customize your rice cakes with additional toppings such as sliced cucumbers, radishes, or a sprinkle of sesame seeds.
- This snack is gluten-free and suitable for vegetarian and vegan diets.

CHAPTER SIX

DESSERTS AND SWEET TREAT

Berry and Coconut Milk Smoothie Bowl

Ingredients:

- 1 cup mixed berries (such as strawberries, blueberries, raspberries)
- 1/2 cup coconut milk (canned, full-fat for creamier texture)
- 1 banana, frozen and sliced
- 1 tablespoon chia seeds (optional, for added thickness)
- Toppings: sliced fresh berries, shredded coconut, granola, sliced almonds, chia seeds, honey or maple syrup (optional)

Instructions:

1. Blend Smoothie Base:
   - In a blender, combine mixed berries, coconut milk, frozen banana slices, and chia seeds if using. Blend until smooth and creamy.

2. Prepare Toppings:
   - While blending, prepare your desired toppings such as sliced fresh berries, shredded coconut, granola, sliced almonds, chia seeds, and honey or maple syrup.

3. Assemble Smoothie Bowl:

- Pour the blended smoothie into a bowl.

4. Add Toppings:
   - Arrange the toppings on top of the smoothie bowl in desired amounts.

5. Serve:
   - Serve immediately and enjoy with a spoon!

Tips:
- Adjust the consistency of the smoothie bowl by adding more or less coconut milk.
- Customize your toppings based on personal preference and dietary needs.
- Experiment with different combinations of berries and other fruits for variety.

Dark Chocolate Avocado Mousse

Ingredients:

- 2 ripe avocados
- 1/4 cup cocoa powder
- 1/4 cup maple syrup or honey (adjust to taste)
- 1 teaspoon vanilla extract
- Pinch of salt
- Optional toppings: shaved dark chocolate, berries, nuts

Instructions:

1. Prepare Avocados:
   - Cut the avocados in half, remove the pits, and scoop the flesh into a food processor or blender.

2. Blend Ingredients:
   - Add cocoa powder, maple syrup or honey, vanilla extract, and a pinch of salt to the food processor or blender with the avocado flesh. Blend until smooth and creamy.

3. Chill (Optional):
   - For a firmer texture, chill the mousse in the refrigerator for at least 30 minutes before serving.

4. Serve:
   - Spoon the dark chocolate avocado mousse into serving dishes.

5. Add Toppings:
   - Garnish with shaved dark chocolate, berries, or nuts if desired.

Tips:
- Ensure avocados are ripe for a smooth texture.
- Adjust sweetness by adding more or less maple syrup or honey.
- Experiment with different toppings such as coconut flakes or a sprinkle of sea salt for added flavor contrast.

Baked Apples with Cinnamon and Walnuts

Ingredients:

- 4 apples (such as Granny Smith or Honeycrisp)
- 1/2 cup chopped walnuts
- 1 tablespoon cinnamon
- 2 tablespoons honey or maple syrup
- 1/4 cup water
- Optional: vanilla ice cream or Greek yogurt (for serving)

Instructions:

1. Prepare Apples:
   - Preheat the oven to 375°F (190°C). Core the apples and cut a small slice off the bottom of each apple so it can stand upright.

2. Stuff Apples:
   - In a bowl, mix together chopped walnuts, cinnamon, and honey or maple syrup. Stuff the mixture into the cored apples.

3. Bake:
   - Place the stuffed apples in a baking dish. Pour water into the bottom of the dish.
   - Bake for 30-40 minutes, or until the apples are tender and the filling is golden brown.

4. Serve:
   - Serve the baked apples warm.

5. Optional:
   - Serve with a scoop of vanilla ice cream or a dollop of Greek yogurt if desired.

Tips:
- Choose firm apples that hold their shape when baked, like Granny Smith or Honeycrisp.
- Check apples for doneness by piercing with a fork; they should be tender.
- Experiment with different nuts such as pecans or almonds for varied textures.

Greek Yogurt with Honey and Berries

Ingredients:

- 1 cup Greek yogurt (plain or flavored)
- 1 tablespoon honey (adjust to taste)
- 1/2 cup mixed berries (such as strawberries, blueberries, raspberries)

Instructions:

1. Prepare Yogurt:
    - Spoon Greek yogurt into a serving bowl.

2. Add Honey and Berries:
    - Drizzle honey over the yogurt.
    - Top with mixed berries.

3. Serve:
    - Serve immediately as a quick and nutritious breakfast or snack.

Tips:
- Use Greek yogurt for a creamy texture and added protein.
- Customize with additional toppings such as granola or nuts for added crunch.
- For a creamier consistency, mix honey into yogurt before adding berries.

Chia Seed Pudding with Mango

Ingredients:

- 1/4 cup chia seeds
- 1 cup almond milk or coconut milk
- 1 tablespoon honey or maple syrup (adjust to taste)
- 1/2 teaspoon vanilla extract
- 1 ripe mango, diced

Instructions:

1. Mix Chia Seeds and Liquid:
   - In a bowl or jar, combine chia seeds, almond milk or coconut milk, honey or maple syrup, and vanilla extract. Stir well to combine.

2. Chill:
   - Cover the bowl or jar and refrigerate for at least 2 hours, or preferably overnight. Stir or shake occasionally within the first hour to prevent clumping.

3. Assemble Pudding:
   - Once the chia seeds have absorbed the liquid and the mixture has thickened to a pudding-like consistency, stir well.

4. Serve:
   - Spoon the chia seed pudding into serving bowls or glasses.

5. Add Mango:

- Top with diced mango before serving.

6. Enjoy Your Chia Seed Pudding with Mango!
  - Serve chilled as a healthy and delicious dessert or snack.

Tips:
- Allow chia seeds to fully absorb liquid for best texture.
- Experiment with different fruits like berries or kiwi for variety.
- Add a sprinkle of cinnamon or nutmeg for extra flavor enhancement.

Banana Oatmeal Cookies

Ingredients

- 2 ripe bananas, mashed
- 1 1/2 cups rolled oats
- 1/4 cup peanut butter or almond butter
- 1/4 cup chocolate chips or raisins (optional)
- 1 teaspoon vanilla extract
- Pinch of cinnamon (optional)

Instructions

1. Preheat Oven:
- Preheat the oven to 350°F (175°C). Line a baking sheet with parchment paper.

2. Mix Ingredients:
- In a bowl, combine mashed bananas, rolled oats, peanut butter or almond butter, chocolate chips or raisins if using, vanilla extract, and cinnamon.

3. Form Cookies:
- Drop spoonfuls of the mixture onto the prepared baking sheet and flatten slightly with a fork.

4. Bake:
- Bake for 15-20 minutes, or until cookies are golden brown and firm.

5. Cool and Serve:- Allow cookies to cool on the baking sheet for 5 minutes before transferring to a wire rack to cool completely.

Tips:
- Customize cookies by adding nuts, dried fruits, or seeds.
- For a softer texture, use ripe bananas.
- Store cookies in an airtight container at room temperature for up to 3 days.

Lemon Blueberry Yogurt Parfait

Ingredients:

- 1 cup Greek yogurt (plain or lemon-flavored)
- 1 cup fresh blueberries
- 1/2 cup granola
- Zest of 1 lemon
- Honey or maple syrup (optional, for sweetness)

Instructions:

1. Layer Ingredients:
- In a glass or bowl, layer Greek yogurt, fresh blueberries, and granola.

2. Repeat Layers:
- Repeat layers until ingredients are used, ending with a sprinkle of granola on top.

3. Add Flavor:
- Sprinkle lemon zest over the top and drizzle with honey or maple syrup if desired.

4. Serve:
- Serve immediately as a refreshing and nutritious dessert or snack.

Tips:
- Use flavored Greek yogurt for added sweetness and variety.

- Substitute blueberries with other berries or fruits like strawberries or raspberries.
- Prepare parfaits ahead of time and refrigerate until ready to serve.

Coconut Macaroons

Ingredients:

- 2 cups shredded coconut (sweetened or unsweetened)
- 1/2 cup sweetened condensed milk
- 1 teaspoon vanilla extract
- 2 egg whites
- Pinch of salt

Instructions:

1. Preheat Oven:
- Preheat the oven to 325°F (160°C). Line a baking sheet with parchment paper.

2. Mix Ingredients:
- In a bowl, combine shredded coconut, sweetened condensed milk, and vanilla extract.

3. Whip Egg Whites:
- In a separate bowl, beat egg whites with a pinch of salt until stiff peaks form.

4. Combine Mixtures:
- Gently fold beaten egg whites into the coconut mixture until well combined.

5. Form Macaroons:

- Drop spoonfuls of the mixture onto the prepared baking sheet, shaping into mounds.

6. Bake:
- Bake for 20-25 minutes, or until macaroons are golden brown on the edges.

7. Cool and Serve:
- Allow macaroons to cool on the baking sheet for 5 minutes before transferring to a wire rack to cool completely.

Tips:
- Dip cooled macaroons in melted chocolate for added decadence.
- Store macaroons in an airtight container at room temperature for up to one week.
- Use unsweetened shredded coconut for a less sweet version.

Peanut Butter Banana Smoothie

Ingredients:

- 2 ripe bananas, peeled and frozen
- 1 cup milk (dairy or almond milk)
- 1/4 cup peanut butter (smooth or crunchy)
- 1 tablespoon honey or maple syrup (optional, for sweetness)
- Ice cubes (optional, for thicker texture)

Instructions:

1. Blend Ingredients:
- In a blender, combine frozen bananas, milk, peanut butter, and honey or maple syrup.

2. Blend Until Smooth:
- Blend until smooth and creamy. Add ice cubes if desired for a thicker texture.

3. Serve:
- Pour into glasses and serve immediately.

Tips:
- Add a handful of spinach or kale for added nutrients.
- Substitute peanut butter with almond butter or sunflower seed butter for variation.
- Garnish with a sprinkle of cocoa powder or chopped nuts for extra flavor.

Mango Coconut Rice Pudding

Ingredients:

- 1 cup cooked white rice
- 1 cup coconut milk
- 1 ripe mango, diced
- 2 tablespoons honey or maple syrup (adjust to taste)
- 1/2 teaspoon vanilla extract
- Pinch of salt
- Toasted coconut flakes (optional, for garnish)

Instructions:

1. Combine Ingredients:
- In a saucepan, combine cooked rice, coconut milk, diced mango, honey or maple syrup, vanilla extract, and a pinch of salt.

2. Simmer:
- Bring mixture to a simmer over medium heat, stirring occasionally.

3. Cook Until Thickened:
- Cook for 15-20 minutes, or until mixture has thickened to desired consistency.

4. Cool:
- Remove from heat and let cool slightly.

5. Serve:
- Spoon rice pudding into serving bowls. Garnish with toasted coconut flakes if desired.

Tips:
- Use leftover cooked rice for a quicker preparation.
- Substitute mango with other fruits like pineapple or berries.
- Serve rice pudding warm or chilled, depending on preference.

CHAPTER SEVEN

MEAL PLANNING TIPS AND SAMPLE MENUS

How To Plan Meals for PCOS

Planning meals for PCOS (Polycystic Ovary Syndrome) involves focusing on nutrient-dense foods that help manage symptoms such as insulin resistance, hormonal imbalances, and weight gain. A well-balanced diet can play a crucial role in alleviating symptoms and promoting overall health. Here's a comprehensive guide to meal planning for PCOS:

1. **Focus on Balanced Macronutrients:**

A balanced diet for PCOS should include a good balance of macronutrients: carbohydrates, proteins, and fats. Opt for complex carbohydrates such as whole grains, legumes, and vegetables, which have a lower glycemic index and help stabilize blood sugar levels. Include lean proteins like poultry, fish, tofu, and legumes to support muscle health and provide satiety. Healthy fats from sources like avocados, nuts, seeds, and olive oil are important for hormone production and overall health.

2. Choose Low-Glycemic Index Foods:

Foods with a low glycemic index (GI) help prevent rapid spikes in blood sugar levels, which can worsen insulin resistance—a common issue in PCOS. Include whole grains like quinoa, brown rice, and oats; legumes such as lentils and chickpeas; and non-starchy vegetables like leafy greens, broccoli, and cauliflower. These foods promote stable blood sugar levels and help manage weight, a key concern for many with PCOS.

3. Prioritize Fiber-Rich Foods:

Fiber plays a crucial role in PCOS management by improving insulin sensitivity and supporting digestive health. Include plenty of fiber-rich foods such as fruits (especially berries), vegetables, whole grains, nuts, seeds, and legumes in your meals. Aim for at least 25-30 grams of fiber per day to promote regularity and help control appetite.

4. Include Anti-Inflammatory Foods:

Chronic inflammation is often associated with PCOS and can exacerbate symptoms. Incorporate anti-inflammatory foods such as fatty fish (salmon, mackerel), turmeric, ginger, berries, leafy greens, and olive oil into your diet. These foods help reduce inflammation and support overall health.

5. Manage Portion Sizes and Caloric Intake:

For weight management, it's important to be mindful of portion sizes and overall caloric intake. While the focus should be on nutrient-dense foods, portion control helps prevent overeating and promotes a healthy weight. Use smaller plates, measure serving sizes, and avoid eating in front of screens to stay aware of portion sizes and avoid mindless eating.

6. Plan Regular Meals and Snacks:

Eating regular meals and snacks throughout the day helps maintain stable blood sugar levels and prevents energy dips. Aim for three balanced meals and two small snacks per day. Include a combination of protein, healthy fats, and fiber in each meal and snack to promote satiety and avoid blood sugar fluctuations.

7. Stay Hydrated:

Adequate hydration is essential for overall health and can support hormone balance. Drink plenty of water throughout the day, and include hydrating foods such as cucumbers, watermelon, and citrus fruits. Limit sugary beverages and caffeine, which can disrupt hormone levels and exacerbate PCOS symptoms.

8. Limit Processed Foods and Added Sugars:

Processed foods, sugary snacks, and beverages can contribute to insulin resistance and weight gain, both of which are common concerns for individuals with PCOS. Limit intake of processed foods, sugary snacks, desserts, and sweetened beverages. Opt for whole, unprocessed foods whenever possible.

9. Plan Ahead and Prep Meals:

Planning meals in advance can help you make healthier choices and avoid impulse eating. Create a weekly meal plan that includes a variety of nutritious foods, and batch cook meals and snacks to save time during the week. Prepare ingredients ahead of time, such as washing and chopping vegetables or cooking grains and proteins, to streamline meal preparation.

10. **Listen to Your Body:**

Pay attention to how different foods make you feel and adjust your diet accordingly. Some individuals with PCOS may benefit from a specific dietary approach, such as low-carbohydrate or Mediterranean-style diets, depending on their symptoms and health goals. Experiment with different foods and meal combinations to find what works best for you.

By following these guidelines and making informed choices about nutrition and meal planning, individuals with PCOS can support their overall health, manage symptoms effectively, and improve quality of life. It's important to consult with a healthcare provider or registered dietitian specializing in PCOS for personalized guidance and support in creating a meal plan that meets individual needs and health goals.

Sample Weekly Meal Plans

Creating a sample weekly meal plan for PCOS (Polycystic Ovary Syndrome) involves selecting nutrient-dense foods that support hormone balance, manage insulin resistance, and promote overall health. Each day should include a balance of complex carbohydrates, lean proteins, healthy fats, and plenty of vegetables and fruits. Here's a comprehensive guide to a sample weekly meal plan for PCOS:

Day 1:

Breakfast: Greek Yogurt Parfait with Berries and Granola
- 1 cup Greek yogurt layered with mixed berries (such as strawberries, blueberries, raspberries) and a sprinkle of granola.
- Use plain Greek yogurt for less added sugar and more protein.

Lunch: Quinoa Salad with Chickpeas and Roasted Vegetables
- Quinoa mixed with chickpeas, roasted vegetables (like bell peppers, zucchini, and cherry tomatoes), fresh herbs, and a drizzle of olive oil and lemon dressing.
- Make extra quinoa for easy meal prep throughout the week.

Dinner: Grilled Salmon with Asparagus and Brown Rice
- Grilled salmon filet served with roasted asparagus and a side of brown rice.
- Salmon provides omega-3 fatty acids, which are beneficial for hormone balance.

Snack: Apple slices with almond butter
- Fresh apple slices dipped in almond butter for a satisfying snack rich in fiber and healthy fats.

Day 2:

Breakfast: Spinach and Feta Egg Muffins
- Egg muffins made with spinach, feta cheese, cherry tomatoes, and herbs, baked until golden.
- Prepare these in advance for a quick and portable breakfast option.

Lunch: Turkey and Vegetable Stir-Fry
- Sliced turkey breast stir-fried with mixed vegetables (like bell peppers, broccoli, and snap peas) in a light soy sauce and ginger sauce, served over quinoa.
- Use lean protein and colorful veggies for a nutrient-packed meal.

Dinner: Lentil and Sweet Potato Curry
- Lentil curry with sweet potatoes, tomatoes, coconut milk, and curry spices, served over brown rice.
- Lentils provide plant-based protein and fiber, beneficial for managing insulin levels.

Snack: Greek yogurt with honey and berries
- Plain Greek yogurt topped with honey and mixed berries for a creamy and antioxidant-rich snack.

Day 3:

Breakfast: Chia Seed Pudding with Mango
- Chia seed pudding made with almond milk, chia seeds, honey, and vanilla extract, topped with diced mango.
- Chia seeds are rich in fiber and omega-3 fatty acids, supporting digestive health and hormone balance.

Lunch: Zucchini Noodles with Pesto and Cherry Tomatoes
- Zucchini noodles (zoodles) tossed with homemade pesto sauce, cherry tomatoes, and pine nuts.
- Zucchini noodles are a low-carb alternative to pasta, ideal for managing insulin resistance.

Dinner: Chicken and Vegetable Soup
- Homemade chicken soup with carrots, celery, onions, and spinach, simmered in a flavorful broth.
- Bone broth provides collagen and nutrients beneficial for gut health and hormone balance.

Snack: Mixed nuts
- A handful of mixed nuts (like almonds, walnuts, and cashews) for a crunchy snack rich in healthy fats and protein.

Day 4:

Breakfast: Berry and Coconut Milk Smoothie Bowl
- Smoothie bowl blended with mixed berries, coconut milk, and topped with granola, shredded coconut, and sliced almonds.
- Smoothie bowls are versatile and can be customized with various toppings for added nutrients.

Lunch: Grilled Chicken Salad with Avocado and Quinoa
- Grilled chicken breast served over a bed of mixed greens, avocado slices, cherry tomatoes, and quinoa, dressed with a light vinaigrette.
- Avocado provides healthy fats and fiber, aiding in hormone regulation.

Dinner: Turkey Meatballs with Marinara Sauce and Spaghetti Squash
- Turkey meatballs simmered in marinara sauce, served over roasted spaghetti squash strands.
- Spaghetti squash is a low-carb alternative to pasta, suitable for managing blood sugar levels.

Snack: Hard-boiled eggs
- Hard-boiled eggs sprinkled with sea salt for a protein-rich snack that helps maintain energy levels.

Day 5:

Breakfast: Green Goddess Hormone Balancing Smoothie
- Smoothie blended with spinach, kale, cucumber, avocado, coconut water, and a squeeze of lemon juice.
- Green smoothies are packed with antioxidants and nutrients that support detoxification and hormone balance.

Lunch: Quinoa Salad Cups with Hummus and Veggies
- Quinoa salad cups filled with hummus, cucumber slices, cherry tomatoes, and olives.
- Quinoa is a gluten-free whole grain that provides fiber and protein, aiding in blood sugar control.

Dinner: Lentil and Vegetable Stuffed Bell Peppers
- Bell peppers stuffed with a mixture of lentils, diced vegetables, herbs, and topped with cheese, baked until tender.
- Bell peppers are rich in vitamin C and antioxidants, supporting immune function and overall health.

Snack: Cottage Cheese with Pineapple
- Cottage cheese topped with fresh pineapple chunks for a protein-packed snack with a touch of sweetness.

Day 6:

Breakfast: Almond Butter Energy Balls
- Energy balls made with almond butter, oats, honey, chia seeds, and dark chocolate chips.
- Energy balls are convenient for on-the-go snacks and provide sustained energy without a sugar crash.

Lunch: Smoked Salmon Cucumber Bites
- Cucumber slices topped with smoked salmon, cream cheese, capers, and dill.
- Smoked salmon provides omega-3 fatty acids, beneficial for heart health and hormone balance.

Dinner: Quinoa Salad with Roasted Chickpeas and Tahini Dressing
- Quinoa salad tossed with roasted chickpeas, mixed greens, cucumber, tomatoes, and drizzled with tahini dressing.
- Tahini (sesame seed paste) adds creamy texture and healthy fats to the salad.

Snack: Edamame
- Steamed edamame pods sprinkled with sea salt for a protein-rich snack that satisfies hunger.

Day 7:

Breakfast: Chocolate Almond Butter Hormone Balancing Smoothie
- Smoothie blended with almond butter, cocoa powder, banana, almond milk, and a scoop of protein powder.
- Add spinach or kale for an extra boost of greens.

Lunch: Stuffed Bell Peppers with Quinoa and Black Beans
- Bell peppers stuffed with quinoa, black beans, corn, tomatoes, and topped with shredded cheese, baked until bubbly.
- Black beans are rich in fiber and protein, aiding in blood sugar control and satiety.

Dinner: Rice Cake with Avocado and Tomato
- Brown rice cakes topped with mashed avocado, sliced tomatoes, and a sprinkle of sea salt and black pepper.
- Brown rice cakes are gluten-free and provide complex carbohydrates for sustained energy.

Snack: Trail Mix
- A homemade trail mix with nuts, seeds, dried fruit (like cranberries or apricots), and dark chocolate chips for a satisfying and nutrient-dense snack.

Additional Tips for Meal Planning:

- **Variety:** Incorporate a variety of colors and textures into your meals to ensure a wide range of nutrients.
- **Hydration:** Drink plenty of water throughout the day to stay hydrated, support digestion, and maintain energy levels.
- **Moderation:** Enjoy treats and indulgences in moderation, focusing on nutrient-dense foods as the foundation of your diet.

- **Preparation:** Prep ingredients and meals ahead of time to save time during busy weekdays and promote healthy eating habits.
- **Consultation:** Consult with a healthcare provider or registered dietitian specializing in PCOS for personalized guidance and adjustments to your meal plan.

By following this sample weekly meal plan and incorporating these tips, individuals with PCOS can support hormone balance, manage symptoms effectively, and improve overall health and well-being. Adjust the meal plan based on personal preferences, dietary needs, and health goals for optimal results.

Tips for Grocery Shopping and Batch Cooking

Grocery shopping and batch cooking are essential strategies for maintaining a healthy diet, especially when managing conditions like PCOS (Polycystic Ovary Syndrome). These practices help ensure you have nutritious meals readily available, streamline meal preparation, and support your overall health goals. Here's a comprehensive guide with tips for grocery shopping and batch cooking tailored for PCOS:

Tips for Grocery Shopping:

1. **Plan Ahead:**

Before heading to the grocery store, take time to plan your meals for the week. Consider your schedule, dietary preferences, and nutritional needs. Create a shopping list based on your meal plan to avoid impulse purchases and ensure you have all the ingredients you need.

2. **Focus on Fresh Produce:**

Fill your cart with a variety of colorful fruits and vegetables. Choose seasonal options when possible for freshness and cost-effectiveness. Opt for leafy greens, berries, cruciferous vegetables (like broccoli and cauliflower), and colorful bell peppers, which are rich in antioxidants and beneficial for hormone balance.

3. **Select Lean Proteins:**

Choose lean sources of protein such as skinless poultry, fish (like salmon and trout), tofu, tempeh, and legumes (such as lentils, chickpeas, and black beans). Protein is essential for muscle repair, hormone production, and satiety, which is important for managing weight and insulin levels.

4. Include Whole Grains:

Stock up on whole grains such as quinoa, brown rice, oats, and whole wheat pasta or bread. These complex carbohydrates have a lower glycemic index compared to refined grains, helping to stabilize blood sugar levels and reduce insulin resistance.

5. Shop the Perimeter:

The perimeter of the grocery store typically contains fresh produce, dairy, and protein sources. Focus on these areas to prioritize nutrient-dense foods and minimize exposure to processed and sugary snacks found in the aisles.

6. Read Labels:

When purchasing packaged foods, read labels carefully to avoid added sugars, trans fats, and artificial ingredients. Look for products with minimal ingredients and choose options labeled as low in added sugars or unsweetened.

7. Healthy Fats:

Include sources of healthy fats in your shopping list such as avocados, nuts (like almonds, walnuts, and pistachios), seeds (such as chia seeds and flaxseeds), and olive oil. These fats are important for hormone synthesis, brain function, and overall health.

8. Dairy and Alternatives:

If you consume dairy, choose low-fat or fat-free options like Greek yogurt or skim milk. Alternatively, opt for dairy-free alternatives like almond milk, coconut yogurt, or soy milk fortified with calcium and vitamin D.

9. Snack Smart:

Choose healthy snacks such as fresh fruit, raw vegetables with hummus or nut butter, Greek yogurt, or homemade energy bars made with nuts and dried fruits. Avoid sugary snacks and processed foods that can contribute to insulin resistance and weight gain.

10. Stay Hydrated:

Don't forget to stock up on water and herbal teas to stay hydrated throughout the day. Limit sugary drinks and caffeinated beverages, which can disrupt hormone balance and contribute to dehydration.

Tips for Batch Cooking:

1. Choose Recipes Wisely:

Select recipes that can be easily scaled up and stored well, such as soups, stews, casseroles, and grain-based salads. Consider one-pot meals or sheet pan dinners for simplified preparation and cleanup.

2. Prep Ingredients:

Before batch cooking, wash, peel, and chop vegetables, marinate proteins, and cook grains or legumes. Prepping ingredients ahead of time saves time during cooking and ensures you have everything ready when you start.

3. Use Storage Containers:

Invest in a variety of storage containers, including glass or BPA-free plastic containers, mason jars, and freezer-safe bags. Portion out meals into individual servings for easy grab-and-go options or family-sized portions for later use.

4. Label and Date:

Label containers with the name of the dish and date of preparation to keep track of freshness. Use masking tape or erasable labels for easy updates.

5. Store Properly:

Refrigerate or freeze batch-cooked meals promptly to maintain freshness and food safety. Divide large batches into smaller portions for quicker thawing and reheating.

6. Rotate Meals:

Plan to consume batch-cooked meals within a few days if refrigerated or within a few months if frozen. Rotate through different dishes to avoid meal fatigue and ensure a balanced diet.

7. Reheat Safely:

When reheating meals, use a microwave or stovetop until heated through. Ensure leftovers reach an internal temperature of 165°F (74°C) to reduce the risk of foodborne illness.

8. Experiment with Freezing:

Some dishes freeze better than others. Experiment with freezing options to determine which meals retain their texture and flavor after thawing.

9. **Maintain Variety:**
Incorporate a variety of flavors and cuisines into your batch-cooked meals to keep meals exciting and enjoyable. Try new recipes or adapt favorite dishes to fit your dietary preferences and nutritional needs.

10. **Enjoy Convenience:**
Batch cooking saves time and effort throughout the week, allowing you to enjoy nutritious meals without the stress of daily cooking. It also helps you resist the temptation of fast food or unhealthy snacks during busy times.

CHAPTER EIGHT

LIFESTYLE TIPS FOR MANAGING PCOS

Importance of Exercise

Exercise plays a crucial role in managing PCOS (Polycystic Ovary Syndrome) by addressing key symptoms such as insulin resistance, weight gain, hormonal imbalances, and overall health. Incorporating regular physical activity into your routine can significantly improve both physical and emotional well-being. Here's a comprehensive look at the importance of exercise in managing PCOS:

1. **Improves Insulin Sensitivity:**
One of the hallmark features of PCOS is insulin resistance, where the body's cells become less responsive to insulin, leading to elevated blood sugar levels. Regular exercise helps improve insulin sensitivity, allowing cells to more efficiently take up glucose from the bloodstream. This helps stabilize blood sugar levels and reduces the risk of developing type 2 diabetes, a common concern for individuals with PCOS.

2. **Aids in Weight Management:**
Weight gain and difficulty losing weight are common challenges for individuals with PCOS. Exercise is essential for

managing weight by increasing calorie expenditure and promoting fat loss, particularly abdominal fat, which is associated with insulin resistance and hormonal imbalances. Combining aerobic exercise (such as brisk walking, jogging, or cycling) with strength training (like weightlifting or bodyweight exercises) can help build muscle mass, boost metabolism, and enhance overall body composition.

3. **Regulates Hormones:**

Hormonal imbalances, including elevated levels of testosterone and irregular menstrual cycles, are prevalent in PCOS. Exercise helps regulate hormones by reducing excessive testosterone production and improving the balance between estrogen and progesterone. This can lead to more regular menstrual cycles and alleviate symptoms such as irregular periods, acne, and unwanted hair growth (hirsutism).

4. **Supports Cardiovascular Health:**

PCOS is associated with an increased risk of cardiovascular disease due to factors like insulin resistance, obesity, and abnormal lipid profiles. Regular exercise improves cardiovascular health by lowering blood pressure, reducing LDL (bad) cholesterol levels, and increasing HDL (good) cholesterol levels. It also enhances vascular function and reduces inflammation, which are critical for reducing cardiovascular risk factors.

5. **Promotes Mental Well-Being:**

Physical activity has profound effects on mental health and well-being. Exercise stimulates the release of endorphins, neurotransmitters that promote feelings of happiness and reduce stress, anxiety, and depression—common issues among individuals with PCOS. Engaging in regular exercise can improve mood, boost self-esteem, and enhance overall quality of life.

6. Enhances Fertility:

Many women with PCOS experience difficulties conceiving due to irregular ovulation or anovulation. Exercise, particularly when combined with a balanced diet and weight management, can improve fertility outcomes by promoting regular menstrual cycles and optimizing reproductive function. For women undergoing fertility treatments, exercise can complement medical interventions and improve the chances of successful conception.

7. Reduces Inflammation:

Chronic inflammation is often elevated in individuals with PCOS and contributes to various symptoms and complications. Exercise has anti-inflammatory effects by reducing levels of inflammatory markers such as C-reactive protein (CRP) and interleukin-6 (IL-6). Regular physical activity also enhances immune function and supports the body's ability to combat inflammation, promoting overall health and well-being.

8. Improves Energy Levels and Sleep Quality:

Fatigue and sleep disturbances are common complaints among individuals with PCOS, often exacerbated by hormonal imbalances and metabolic issues. Exercise helps improve energy levels by enhancing mitochondrial function and oxygen delivery to tissues. It also promotes better sleep quality by regulating circadian rhythms and reducing symptoms of insomnia, leading to more restorative sleep patterns.

9. **Builds Strong Bones and Muscles:**

Regular weight-bearing exercises such as walking, jogging, dancing, and strength training help build and maintain bone density, reducing the risk of osteoporosis—a concern for women with PCOS, especially those with irregular menstrual cycles. Strength training exercises also build muscle mass and strength, which supports joint stability, posture, and overall physical function.

10. **Promotes Long-Term Health and Well-Being:**

Adopting a consistent exercise routine promotes long-term health benefits beyond managing PCOS symptoms. Regular physical activity reduces the risk of chronic diseases such as diabetes, cardiovascular disease, and certain cancers. It also fosters healthy habits, enhances resilience to stress, and improves overall life expectancy.

Incorporating Exercise into Your Routine:

To maximize the benefits of exercise for managing PCOS, aim for at least 150 minutes of moderate-intensity aerobic activity, such as brisk walking or cycling, per week, or 75 minutes of vigorous-intensity activity, such as running or swimming. Include strength training exercises two to three times per week to build muscle and improve metabolism. Choose activities that you enjoy and can sustain over time, whether it's group fitness classes, outdoor activities, or home workouts.

Always consult with a healthcare provider or certified fitness professional before starting a new exercise program, especially if you have any existing health conditions or concerns. They can provide personalized recommendations based on your medical history, fitness level, and specific goals to help you safely and effectively manage PCOS through regular physical activity.

Stress Management Techniques

Managing stress is crucial for individuals with PCOS (Polycystic Ovary Syndrome) as stress can exacerbate symptoms and impact overall well-being. Implementing effective stress management techniques can help reduce the physiological and psychological impact of stress, improve hormonal balance, and enhance quality of life. Here's an in-depth exploration of stress management techniques for individuals managing PCOS:

1. **Mindfulness Meditation:**

Mindfulness meditation involves focusing on the present moment without judgment, which can help reduce stress and anxiety associated with PCOS symptoms. Regular practice improves emotional regulation, enhances self-awareness, and promotes relaxation responses that counteract the body's stress response.

2. **Deep Breathing Exercises:**

Deep breathing exercises, such as diaphragmatic breathing or box breathing, activate the body's relaxation response and decrease stress hormones like cortisol. These techniques can be practiced anywhere and help restore calm during stressful situations.

3. **Progressive Muscle Relaxation (PMR):**

PMR involves tensing and then relaxing each muscle group in the body systematically, promoting physical relaxation and reducing tension. It helps alleviate muscle stiffness and promotes overall relaxation, which can be particularly beneficial for individuals experiencing physical symptoms of stress.

4. **Yoga and Tai Chi:**
Yoga and Tai Chi combine physical postures, breathing exercises, and meditation to improve flexibility, balance, and mental focus. These mind-body practices reduce stress levels, improve mood, and enhance overall well-being by integrating physical movement with mindfulness techniques.

5. **Regular Exercise:**
Physical activity not only improves physical health but also plays a vital role in reducing stress and anxiety. Exercise stimulates the production of endorphins, neurotransmitters that promote feelings of well-being and happiness. Engaging in regular exercise routines such as walking, jogging, dancing, or yoga can effectively alleviate stress and improve mood.

6. **Journaling:**
Writing down thoughts, feelings, and experiences in a journal can provide clarity, insight, and emotional release. Journaling allows individuals to process emotions, identify stress triggers, and develop coping strategies. It serves as a personal tool for self-reflection and stress management.

7. **Healthy Lifestyle Habits:**
Adopting healthy lifestyle habits such as adequate sleep, balanced nutrition, and limiting caffeine and alcohol intake can significantly reduce stress levels. Prioritizing self-care activities, establishing regular sleep patterns, and consuming a

nutrient-dense diet support overall health and resilience to stress.

8. Social Support:

Maintaining strong social connections and seeking support from friends, family, or support groups can buffer the impact of stress. Sharing experiences, seeking advice, and receiving empathy from others facing similar challenges can provide emotional validation and reduce feelings of isolation.

9. Time Management and Prioritization:

Effective time management and prioritization techniques, such as creating daily schedules or using task management tools, help individuals with PCOS manage responsibilities and reduce stress associated with feeling overwhelmed. Setting realistic goals and breaking tasks into manageable steps promote a sense of control and accomplishment.

10. Professional Counseling or Therapy:

Seeking professional counseling or therapy can be beneficial for individuals experiencing chronic stress, anxiety, or depression related to PCOS. Cognitive-behavioral therapy (CBT), mindfulness-based stress reduction (MBSR), or other therapeutic approaches can provide personalized strategies for managing stress, improving coping skills, and enhancing overall emotional well-being.

Incorporating Stress Management Techniques:

To effectively manage stress with PCOS, integrate these techniques into your daily routine based on personal preferences and needs. Experiment with different methods to identify which approaches are most effective for reducing stress and improving overall quality of life. Consistency and patience are key as you develop habits that support emotional resilience and empower you to better manage the challenges associated with PCOS. Consulting with healthcare providers or mental health professionals can provide additional guidance and support tailored to your individual circumstances and goals.

Sleep and PCOS

Sleep plays a crucial role in managing PCOS (Polycystic Ovary Syndrome) by influencing hormone regulation, metabolic function, and overall well-being. Individuals with PCOS often experience sleep disturbances, which can exacerbate symptoms and impact health outcomes. Implementing effective sleep hygiene practices and addressing sleep-related issues are essential for managing PCOS effectively.

Adequate sleep is essential for regulating hormones involved in PCOS, including insulin, cortisol, and reproductive hormones such as estrogen, progesterone, and testosterone. Disrupted sleep patterns or insufficient sleep can lead to hormonal imbalances, exacerbating symptoms such as insulin resistance, irregular menstrual cycles, and fertility issues.

Sleep deprivation or poor sleep quality can contribute to metabolic disturbances commonly associated with PCOS, such as obesity, insulin resistance, and dyslipidemia. Quality sleep supports metabolic processes by promoting glucose regulation, reducing inflammation, and optimizing energy metabolism, all of which are critical for managing PCOS symptoms and reducing long-term health risks.

Adequate sleep is important for weight management, as it influences appetite regulation and food cravings. Sleep deprivation can disrupt the balance of hunger hormones like leptin and ghrelin, leading to increased appetite, overeating, and weight gain—factors that can exacerbate insulin resistance and hormonal imbalances in individuals with PCOS.

Sleep plays a vital role in emotional regulation and mental health. Chronic sleep disturbances are associated with increased risk of anxiety, depression, and mood disorders, which are common among individuals with PCOS. Improving sleep quality can enhance mood stability, reduce stress levels, and promote overall emotional well-being.

Maintaining regular sleep-wake cycles supports healthy circadian rhythms, which regulate physiological processes such as hormone secretion, metabolism, and immune function. Disrupted circadian rhythms, often observed in individuals with irregular sleep patterns or shift work, can adversely affect health outcomes and exacerbate PCOS symptoms.

Sleep influences reproductive health and fertility outcomes in individuals with PCOS. Irregular sleep patterns or sleep disorders may disrupt menstrual cycles, ovulation, and reproductive hormone balance, impacting fertility potential. Prioritizing consistent and restorative sleep supports reproductive function and enhances chances of conceiving for individuals planning pregnancy.

Strategies for Improving Sleep Quality with PCOS:

1. Establish a Consistent Sleep Schedule:
Aim for a regular sleep-wake cycle by going to bed and waking up at the same time each day, even on weekends. Consistency helps regulate circadian rhythms and promotes better sleep quality over time.

2. Create a Relaxing Bedtime Routine:
Develop calming pre-sleep rituals such as reading, gentle stretching, or taking a warm bath to signal to your body that it's time to wind down. Avoid stimulating activities and electronics close to bedtime, as blue light exposure can interfere with melatonin production.

3. Optimize Sleep Environment:
Create a conducive sleep environment that is cool, dark, and quiet. Invest in a comfortable mattress and pillows that support restful sleep. Use blackout curtains or a sleep mask to minimize light exposure that can disrupt sleep.

4. Practice Good Sleep Hygiene:
Adopt practices that promote better sleep hygiene, such as limiting caffeine and alcohol intake, avoiding heavy meals close to bedtime, and creating a comfortable sleep environment. Maintain a relaxing bedtime routine and avoid screens that emit blue light.

5. Manage Stress and Anxiety:
Stress and anxiety can significantly impact sleep quality. Incorporate stress management techniques such as mindfulness

meditation, deep breathing exercises, or yoga into your daily routine to promote relaxation and reduce nighttime stress.

6. Limit Daytime Naps:

While short naps can be beneficial, especially for combating daytime fatigue, avoid long or irregular naps that can disrupt nighttime sleep patterns. If you need to nap, aim for 20-30 minutes earlier in the day to minimize interference with nighttime sleep.

7. Regular Physical Activity:

Engage in regular physical activity, but avoid vigorous exercise close to bedtime as it may be stimulating. Moderate aerobic exercise, such as walking or swimming, can promote better sleep quality and overall health in individuals with PCOS.

8. Seek Professional Support:

If sleep disturbances persist despite implementing these strategies, consult with a healthcare provider or sleep specialist. They can assess potential underlying factors contributing to sleep problems and recommend personalized interventions or treatments to improve sleep quality and overall well-being.

By prioritizing sleep and implementing these strategies, individuals with PCOS can support hormone balance, metabolic health, emotional well-being, and overall quality of life. Consistent efforts to improve sleep hygiene and address sleep-related issues contribute to effective management of PCOS symptoms and promote long-term health outcomes.

CHAPTER NINE

RESOURCES AND FURTHER READING

Recommended Books and Websites

Finding reliable resources, whether in books or online, is crucial for individuals managing PCOS (Polycystic Ovary Syndrome) to access accurate information, guidance, and support. Here's a comprehensive guide to recommended books and websites that provide valuable insights into PCOS management, nutrition, lifestyle recommendations, and emotional support:

Recommended Books:

1. "The PCOS Workbook: Your Guide to Complete Physical and Emotional Health" by Angela Grassi, MS, RDN, LDN

This comprehensive workbook offers practical strategies for managing PCOS through nutrition, exercise, and emotional well-being. It includes meal plans, recipes, and worksheets to support individuals in developing personalized lifestyle changes.

2. **"PCOS Diet for the Newly Diagnosed: Your All-In-One Guide to Eliminating PCOS Symptoms with the Insulin Resistance Diet" by Tara Spencer**

Tara Spencer provides a straightforward approach to managing PCOS symptoms through diet and lifestyle modifications. The book includes meal plans, recipes, and tips for navigating insulin resistance and hormonal imbalances.

3. **"The PCOS Solution: An Evidence-Based Natural Approach to Healing PCOS" by Dr. Nirali Patel, ND**

Dr. Nirali Patel offers an integrative approach to PCOS treatment, combining naturopathic medicine, nutrition, and lifestyle modifications. The book covers hormone balance, fertility concerns, and holistic strategies for managing PCOS symptoms.

4. **"8 Steps to Reverse Your PCOS: A Proven Program to Reset Your Hormones, Repair Your Metabolism, and Restore Your Fertility" by Dr. Fiona McCulloch, ND**

Dr. Fiona McCulloch provides a comprehensive guide to reversing PCOS symptoms through evidence-based strategies. The book explores diet, supplements, stress management, and personalized treatment plans for hormone balance and reproductive health.

5. **"The PCOS Plan: Prevent and Reverse Polycystic Ovary Syndrome through Diet and Fasting" by Hillary Wright, MEd, RDN**

Hillary Wright introduces a science-backed approach to PCOS management through dietary modifications and intermittent fasting. The book includes meal plans, recipes, and guidance on optimizing metabolic health and hormone balance.

Recommended Websites:

1. **PCOS Nutrition Center**
   Website:
[pcosnutrition.com](https://www.pcosnutrition.com)

The PCOS Nutrition Center, founded by Angela Grassi, provides evidence-based nutrition information, recipes, and resources for managing PCOS through diet and lifestyle changes. It offers personalized consultations and online courses for individuals seeking guidance.

2. **PCOS Diva**

Website: pcosdiva.com

PCOS Diva, created by Amy Medling, offers holistic strategies for living well with PCOS. The website features articles, podcasts, recipes, and lifestyle tips focusing on nutrition, exercise, mindfulness, and emotional well-being.

3. **Soul Cysters**

Website: [soulcysters.com](https://www.soulcysters.com)

Soul Cysters is an online community and resource hub for women with PCOS. It provides forums for support, discussions on PCOS-related topics, treatment options, and personal stories from individuals navigating their PCOS journey.

4. **The Hormone Health Network**
   Website: [hormone.org](https://www.hormone.org)

The Hormone Health Network offers reliable information on hormonal disorders, including PCOS. It provides educational resources, articles, and tools for understanding hormone-related conditions, treatment options, and lifestyle management.

5. **Mayo Clinic**

   Website: [mayoclinic.org](https://www.mayoclinic.org)

   The Mayo Clinic website provides comprehensive information on PCOS, including symptoms, causes, diagnosis, and treatment options. It offers reliable medical insights, lifestyle recommendations, and patient resources for managing PCOS effectively.

These books and websites offer valuable resources and support for individuals seeking information on PCOS management, nutrition, lifestyle modifications, and emotional well-being. They provide evidence-based insights, practical strategies, and community support to empower individuals in effectively managing PCOS and improving overall health outcomes.

Support Groups and Online Communities

Finding support groups and online communities can provide invaluable emotional support, shared experiences, and practical advice for individuals managing PCOS (Polycystic Ovary Syndrome). Here's a guide to recommended support groups and online communities dedicated to PCOS:

Recommended Support Groups and Online Communities:

1. **Soul Cysters**
   - Website: [soulcysters.com](https://www.soulcysters.com)
   - Soul Cysters is a longstanding online community for women with PCOS. It offers forums for discussions on PCOS symptoms, treatments, lifestyle strategies, and emotional support. Members share personal experiences, offer advice, and connect with others facing similar challenges.

2. **PCOS Awareness Association**
   - Website: pcosaa.org
   - The PCOS Awareness Association provides resources, educational materials, and support for individuals affected by PCOS. It hosts online support groups, webinars, and community events to raise awareness and empower individuals with PCOS to advocate for their health.

3. **PCOS Challenge: The National Polycystic Ovary Syndrome Association**
   - Website: pcoschallenge.org

- PCOS Challenge is a nonprofit organization dedicated to raising awareness about PCOS and providing support for individuals affected by the condition. It offers online support groups, educational resources, advocacy initiatives, and community events to empower individuals with PCOS.

4. **Reddit PCOS Community**
   - **Subreddit: [r/PCOS](https://www.reddit.com/r/PCOS/)**
   - The PCOS subreddit on Reddit provides a platform for individuals to share stories, ask questions, and discuss various aspects of PCOS management. Members offer support, share personal experiences, and provide insights into treatment options, lifestyle changes, and coping strategies.

5. **My PCOS Team**
   - Website: [mypcosteam.com](https://www.mypcosteam.com)
   - My PCOS Team is an online social network and support community for individuals with PCOS. Members can connect with others, share updates, ask questions, and offer support to fellow members navigating their PCOS journey. The platform also features resources and educational content related to PCOS management.

Benefits of Joining Support Groups and Online Communities:

- Emotional Support: Engaging with others who understand the challenges of living with PCOS can provide emotional validation, reduce feelings of isolation, and offer encouragement during difficult times.

- Shared Experiences: Connecting with individuals who share similar experiences allows for the exchange of practical tips, personal insights, and coping strategies for managing PCOS symptoms effectively.

- Information and Resources: Support groups and online communities often provide access to reliable information, educational resources, and updates on PCOS research, treatment options, and lifestyle recommendations.

- Empowerment and Advocacy: Joining a community of individuals affected by PCOS can empower individuals to advocate for their health, participate in awareness campaigns, and access resources to better navigate their PCOS journey.

- Community Engagement: Participating in discussions, attending virtual events, and contributing to community initiatives foster a sense of belonging and mutual support among members.

Getting Involved:

To benefit fully from support groups and online communities:

- Join Discussions: Participate actively in discussions, ask questions, and share your experiences to contribute to the community and gain insights from others.

- Attend Events: Take advantage of virtual events, webinars, and workshops hosted by support groups to learn from experts, connect with peers, and stay informed about PCOS-related topics.

- Seek Support: Reach out for support when needed, whether for emotional encouragement, practical advice, or navigating treatment options. Utilize the community as a resource for addressing concerns and accessing relevant information.

CONCLUSION

In navigating the complexities of PCOS (Polycystic Ovary Syndrome), we've explored a multifaceted approach encompassing nutrition, lifestyle modifications, stress management, and community support. PCOS affects millions of individuals worldwide, presenting unique challenges that extend beyond physical health to encompass emotional well-being and quality of life. Throughout this book, we've delved into evidence-based strategies, practical tips, and empowering insights aimed at empowering individuals to effectively manage their PCOS journey.

Central to managing PCOS is adopting a balanced and supportive diet. We've emphasized the importance of nutrient-dense foods, including whole grains, lean proteins, fruits, vegetables, and healthy fats. These choices not only help regulate blood sugar levels and improve insulin sensitivity but also support hormonal balance and overall metabolic health. Through recipes, meal plans, and nutritional guidelines, we've provided tools to make informed dietary choices tailored to individual needs and preferences.

Beyond diet, lifestyle modifications play a pivotal role in PCOS management. Regular physical activity has emerged as a cornerstone, aiding in weight management, hormone regulation, and stress reduction. Incorporating exercise routines that combine aerobic activities and strength training not only supports physical health but also enhances mental well-being and resilience. We've explored the benefits of stress management techniques, sleep hygiene practices, and mindfulness strategies to mitigate the impact of stress on PCOS symptoms and overall health outcomes.

Navigating PCOS can be daunting, but connecting with others facing similar challenges can provide invaluable support, validation, and encouragement. We've highlighted the importance of joining support groups and online communities where individuals can share experiences, exchange information, and find solidarity. These platforms offer a safe space to discuss concerns, access resources, and foster a sense of community that empowers individuals to advocate for their health and well-being.

Each person's journey with PCOS is unique, influenced by factors such as genetics, lifestyle, and individual health goals. Throughout this book, we've emphasized the significance of personalized care and treatment plans tailored to individual needs. Whether exploring treatment options with healthcare providers, experimenting with dietary adjustments, or incorporating lifestyle changes, empowering informed decision-making is essential for managing PCOS effectively
As research and understanding of PCOS continue to evolve, so too do our approaches to managing and supporting individuals affected by this syndrome. The journey to managing PCOS is ongoing, requiring dedication, resilience, and a commitment to holistic health. By embracing the principles outlined in this book—nutrition, lifestyle modifications, stress management,

and community support—we can navigate the complexities of PCOS with confidence and empowerment.

In conclusion, managing PCOS is not just about alleviating symptoms but about optimizing health and well-being across all facets of life. By adopting a proactive and holistic approach that integrates nutrition, lifestyle modifications, stress management, and community support, individuals with PCOS can enhance their quality of life and empower themselves to thrive. This book serves as a comprehensive guide and companion on your PCOS journey, providing tools, resources, and insights to support you every step of the way. Together, we can continue to foster awareness, advocate for better care, and empower individuals with PCOS to lead healthier, fulfilling lives.

As you embark on your path forward, remember that you are not alone. With knowledge, support, and perseverance, you have the ability to navigate PCOS with resilience and optimism. Here's to embracing health, empowerment, and a brighter future ahead.

www.ingramcontent.com/pod-product-compliance
Lightning Source LLC
Chambersburg PA
CBHW031419210526
45464CB00005B/1959